NATURAL HEALTHCARE AT HOME

Natural Healthcare at Home

Doctor Mum's Quick Reference Guide

Kathy Duerr

New Age Books

ISBN: 81-7822-017-2

First Indian Edition: 2001

First Published in 2000 under the title
"Doctor Mum's Quick Reference Guide to Natural Healthcare at Home"
by Findhorn Press, U.K.

Disclaimer:
This book is sold with the understanding that the author and publisher are not liable for the misconception or misuse of the information provided. The author and publisher shall have neither liability nor responsibility to any person or entity with respect to any loss, damage, or injury caused or alleged to be caused directly or indirectly by the information contained in this book. The information in this book is in no way intended as a substitute for medical counseling.

Published by
NEW AGE BOOKS
A-44 Naraina Phase I
New Delhi-110 028 (INDIA)
Email: info@newagebooksindia.com
Website: www.newagebooksindia.com

For Sale in Indian Subcontinent Only

Printed in India
at Shri Jainendra Press
A-45 Naraina Phase-I New Delhi-110 028

To my three children,

Emily, Abani, and Sean,

who have successfully responded

to these treatments.

Table of Contents

Foreword

This is a great book, concise, and accurate. *Doctor Mom's Quick Reference Guide to Natural Healthcare at Home* is just what it says it is, a quick reference guide to the treatment of the most common conditions that affect babies, children, and even adults. Every home should have this book. I have authored a few books on the care of babies and children and have gone to pedantic and boring lengths, afraid that I might leave something out. Kathy Duerr gives the reader the essentials. Mothers and caretakers of children can be assured that Kathy has tried all these remedies on her own three children with great success. The best recommendation I can make for the book is that these remedies work.

As a pediatrician, before I learned about natural ways of assuaging disease, I gave antibiotics for most throat and ear infections. This only seemed to allow these infections to recur. I was not letting the child's immune system learn from infection. Not a thing was said in my medical school about these natural methods. Thanks for helping me, Doctor Mom.

Lendon Smith, M.D.
Author of *How to Raise a Healthy Child*

Acknowledgments

My introduction to alternative medicine began with the study of medicinal plants. My first mentors were those in the field of botanical medicine: Olinka Hardy then age 72, a Native American, and Marie Wilks, age 80, Italian born and trained in the Bio-dynamic method of agriculture. These old women, who grew and used herbs as a way of life, taught me the many gifts that appear in this book. They schooled me in the fine art of herbal preparations, such as salves, tinctures, poultices, and compresses, and in how to use them as medicine. Alan Chadwick, a master gardener trained in Bio-dynamic French intensive gardening taught me the advantages of growing plants without chemicals and the healing power of food, flowers, and herbs.

A special thank you to Bob Grunnet for introducing me to the wonders of homeopathy and teaching me to trust myself as a healer. To doctors Bruce Canvasser, N.D. and John Collins, N.D. for the support and confidence bestowed upon me in consultations, many thanks.

Introduction

At the age of 22, I became aware that there was a healer inside of me, struggling for a way of expression. My initiation into healing was through gardening. As the plants in my garden called and spoke to me, I found a love I did not know I was capable of. In no time at all I was growing herbs, unaware as to how powerful they were and how they would shape a life for me that I live to this day. Following a strong desire to improve my lifestyle by eating organic food and growing my own plants for medicine, I began planting a little garden. As I learned to use plants for healing, I realized that I wanted to care for my own family without depending on pharmaceutical preparations. Even then it was common knowledge that over-the-counter products can be risky, many times causing side effects that have to be dealt with on top of the original symptoms.

I undertook the task of educating myself in the ways of the barefoot doctor, including growing, harvesting, and preparing plants for medicine. Not long after I began this journey, I started having babies of my own and began to practice what I was learning. I was fearless and self-assured, using plain, simple, old-time remedies that worked every time. All three of my children were born at home with midwives, using natural medicine. We used herbs, homeopathy, and hydrotherapy during my pregnancies and births. It is possible to care safely for your family using the natural medicines recommended in this book and to feel comfortable and confident while doing so. Trust yourself as a mother to feel the needs of your child. Using these simple remedies will help you regain your inner gift of healing. This book is my gift of support to all the mothers who prefer not to resort to over-the-counter drugs and pharmaceuticals for the everyday medical care of their families.

Be sure to visit Doctor Mom's website on

www.drmomsnaturalmedicine.com

Part 1

FOUNDATIONS
OF
GOOD HEALTH

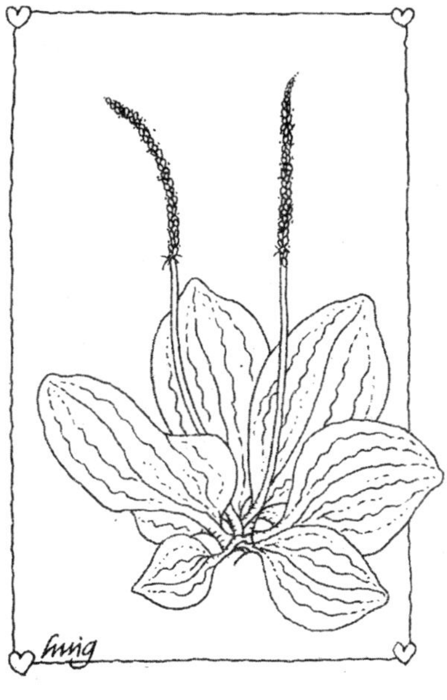

Choosing to use natural medicine gives you the opportunity to make a profound difference in the health and well-being of your child. It is one area where you can actually do something that will have a positive effect on your child's future. Currently everyone is born into a toxic world that we seemingly have no control over. The water, air, and earth are loaded with various levels of pollution that affect the health of our children. Our homes, offices, and schools are contaminated with toxic building materials. Everyday we come in contact with many substances that weaken our immune system and adversely affect our health. These areas of life are difficult to control, and we are at the mercy of our environment.

By using natural medicine in the form of food, herbs, homeopathy, and water treatments you can actually help your children to build strong bodies that are more resistant to disease. You can even prevent disease with the regular use of natural medicines. Herbs make the body stronger, as does healthy food, and homeopathy triggers the body's own defense mechanisms to heal itself. Homeopathy is safe, very effective, inexpensive, extremely easy to use, and kids love it. Water therapies also boost the immune system by increasing circulation and blood flow, helping the body to cleanse and heal itself, thus creating a strong body where infectious organisms are unable to live.

The use of antibiotics and other drugs weaken the body by killing beneficial organisms and cause side effects. They do nothing to strengthen the body's own defense mechanisms. Natural treatments support and stimulate the immune system creating a healthier body that is able to fight infection and prevent serious and chronic disease.

You can help prevent disease and protect your child merely by paying attention to diet and preparing natural, healthy food on a regular basis. Setting up healthy habits in young children makes a big difference. Teach your children to drink water when thirsty instead of sugar-laden, artificially flavored drinks. It takes a little more energy and forethought in the beginning, but the outcome will be well worth the effort.

When a child shows the first signs of becoming ill, have her drink a glass of purified water. Water is a great healer that many of us have forgotten. Our lives have become so complicated that something as simple as a glass of water is far from our minds. Water soothes, cleanses, and refreshes us when we are weary and feeling out of sorts. Many times, just by increasing water intake, one will become well again. Start your baby right by getting into the habit of giving her water in a bottle, not just milk or juice all the time. Don't forget to give your children more water on hot days.

Herbal teas are a great alternative to the usual sugary drinks. Make the tea in the morning by placing two tea bags in a quart jar of boiling water. Let the tea steep for five minutes, remove the tea bags and add a little honey. Set the tea in the refrigerator until cold. Serve to the kids on a sunny afternoon. Add some lemon, lime, or orange slices for a festive-looking beverage. Sprigs of lemon balm, lavender, or mint give a subtle flavor and a visual complement. These are good habits to start your child on early. Then when she gets sick with a cold or flu, she will welcome the idea of a familiar drink.

Give warm, gentle herb teas with a little lemon and honey at the onset of illness. Never give an infant or child hot tea. The temperature of the tea should be the same as the temperature of a bottle of warm milk. This is soothing and comforting to children. Most babies and children like teas that have a mild flavor. Start them on spearmint, peppermint, chamomile, or hibiscus, or any combinations that include these herbs.

Begin giving your baby diluted herb tea in his bottle at age two months. Whenever you give your child a bottle, always hold him in your arms rather than laying him down alone with the bottle propped up on a pillow. I know you are very busy with so many things to do and are always looking for ways to get a little more time to yourself, but there is nothing more relaxing than to take a moment with your child while giving him a bottle, making eye contact and drifting off for a bit in the mid-afternoon. Both of you benefit from these quiet, nurturing moments. Take advantage of these opportunities whenever you can. Infancy is precious, shortlived, and gone before you know it. You will never regret spending more time with your children.

This guide is intended to assist the mother in relieving her children's discomfort in acute medical conditions. Since the beginning of time it has been a mother's role to provide healthcare for her family. It is natural and safe to use common, simple remedies while caring for your children at home, and to feel comfortable doing so. Always consult a physician in cases of chronic illness, severe distress, or any time your parental instincts tell you to do so.

Home Medicinary

Being prepared is the most important aspect of giving proper and effective care. There is nothing worse than being unable to help your child when on a Sunday evening he starts to complain of a common ailment, and you know a simple treatment, but you haven't the remedy on hand and the stores are closed. In many instances early treatment can stop the development of a full-blown disease. Make it your first priority to put together the following home medicinary and other necessary items. I have tried to make this list brief yet adequate, so as not to overwhelm the newcomer to natural medicine.

SUPPLIES

ACE BANDAGES

BAND-AIDS: In a variety of sizes, including butterfly band-aids.

COTTON GAUZE AND TAPE

BAKING SODA

HAND TOWELS: Three of thin cotton.

MUSIC TAPES OF CHILDREN'S LULLABIES: Better yet, learn some simple lullabies to sing to your children at any time, and especially when they are sick.

PACKS: Thick plastic bags filled with a gel-like substance that can withstand both hot and cold temperature. Keep one in the freezer to be used as a cold pack and one in the cupboard to be warmed up in hot water and used the same as a hot water bottle.

ROCKING CHAIR: Holding your child while rocking is very healing. It's so easy for mothers to forget this healing technique with all the modern-day paraphernalia, such as baby swings, strollers, and rocking infant seats. Your energy, your voice, your breath, and your heartbeat nurture, heal, and stimulate the growth and health of your child every time you hold him.

OINTMENTS, GELS, AND CREAMS

ALOE VERA: Usually comes in a gel. Cooling and soothing for cuts, scrapes, or minor burns. It is especially healing for sunburn. If you have an aloe vera plant of three years or older you can use the plant itself. Cut a leaf at the base of the plant and peel off the outer skin to expose the gel-like substance and swab the area generously with it several times a day. Store the remaining leaf in a plastic bag and refrigerate until you want to reuse it.

ARNICA: For sprains, bruises, or trauma to head or joints. ***Do not*** use on any injury where the skin is broken.

CALENDULA: Good for any open wound where the skin has been broken.

COMFREY: For bruises, sprains, twisted ankles and swelling, and for cuts and scrapes after the bleeding has stopped.

OILS

CASTOR OIL: Used to make compresses for healing all types of internal inflammation.

CITRONELLA OIL: Used as an insect repellent, especially for mosquitoes.

MULLEIN OIL: Used specifically for earaches and minor ear infections.

OLIVE OIL: Used as a base to mix with powdered or crushed herbs. Also good for massaging the feet of a fussy child or infant.

HERBS IN BULK

In most cases, an ounce of each of these herbs will be plenty to have on hand. I recommend buying small amounts and replacing them regularly to ensure freshness. You can determine the freshness of herbs by paying attention to vibrancy of color and a strong fragrance. It is advisable to replace or replenish your herbs yearly. *Do not store bulk herbs in direct sunlight.*

There are several ways to administer botanicals to children. A very young or uncooperative child can be given a foot bath. Find a bowl that is large enough for your child to put her feet in comfortably. Prepare the foot bath by placing the dried herb in a little cotton sock or muslin bag, and pour boiling water over it. Let it steep for about five minutes, and then add some cool water. The water should be warm (be careful it's not too hot!) and deep enough to cover her ankles when she places her feet in the bowl. This is a nice time for you and your child to enjoy a cup of herb tea together.

If the child is too young or too ill to sit up, mix about a teaspoon of the powdered herb in a tablespoon of olive oil, and rub the mixture on the bottoms of her feet. Put a clean pair of socks on her and put her to bed. The herbs will be better absorbed if you can soak the child's feet in some warm water for a few minutes before massaging in the herbal mixture. Dry the foot off first and then rub in the olive oil and herbs. This is a comfortable, non-invasive, enjoyable way to give your baby or child an herbal remedy.

You can also administer herbs in a full-body bath. Fill a small cotton sock or muslin bag with the herbs indicated, and steep them in the bath as you would in a cup of tea. Bathe your child in the herb-steeped water for at least ten minutes. The temperature of the water should be the same as for normal bathing.

KEEP THE FOLLOWING HERBS IN DRIED FORM:

CALENDULA FLOWERS: Internally used as an infusion for stomach cramps, diarrhea, ulcers, fever, and abscesses. Externally used in ointment, tea, cream, or tincture form for open wounds, bruises, sprains, sores, boils, warts, chickenpox, and skin rashes.

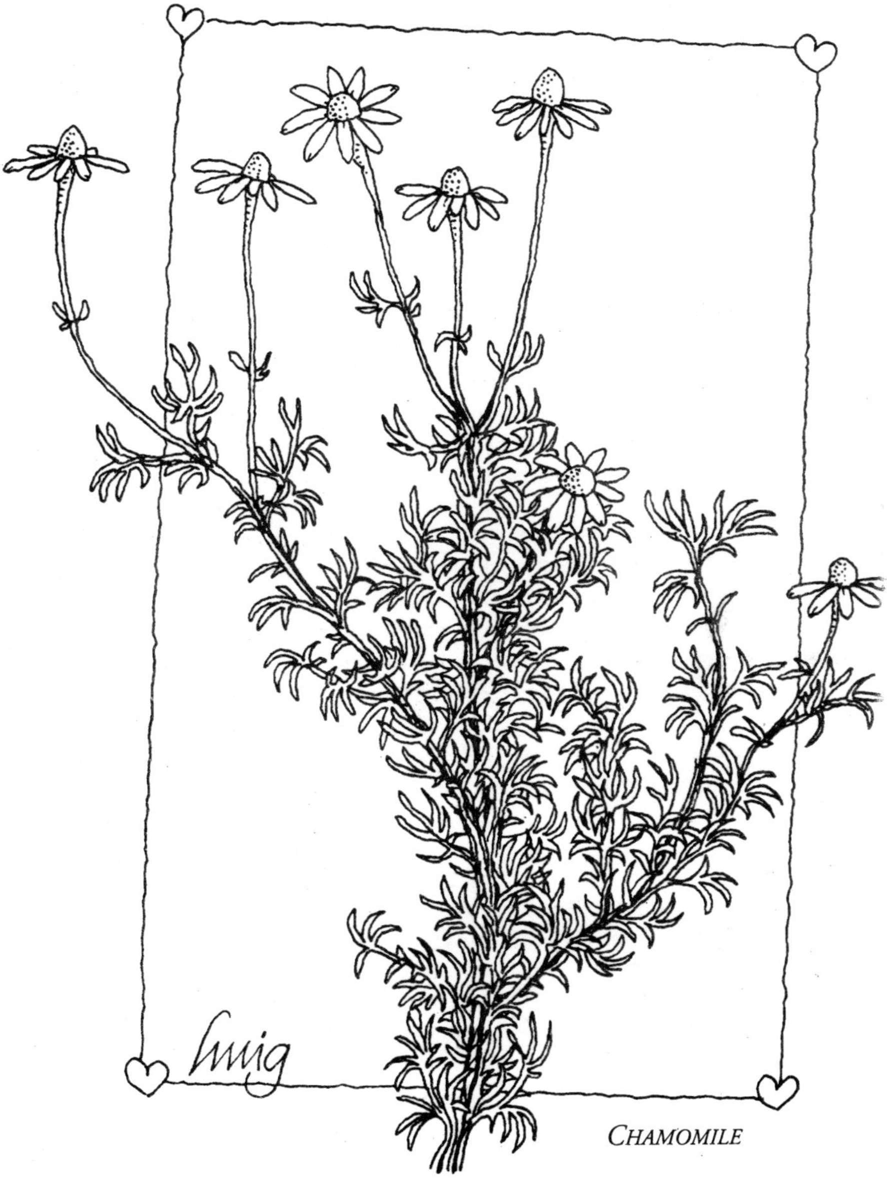

CHAMOMILE

CHAMOMILE FLOWERS: Internally used as an infusion for insomnia, as a calmative, for stomachache and teething, and for facilitating bowel movement. Externally for inflammation of mucus tissue, teething, and as a relaxing, calming bath for the irritable child.

COMFREY LEAVES AND ROOT POWDER (keep separate): Internally used as an infusion of the leaves for most stomach and digestive disorders, ulcers, colitis, and broken bones. Externally the root powder is used for the care of the umbilical cord and for wounds. The leaves are prepared as a poultice for broken bones, sprains, soft tissue injuries, bites, and boils.

GARLIC CLOVES (fresh, not dried): Internally given as capsules of garlic oil or prepared in food, used as a natural antibiotic for the prevention and early treatment of colds, flu, and inflammatory disease. Externally, crushed garlic mixed with olive oil is applied as a paste to the bottom of a child's feet for the prevention and treatment of colds, flu, sore throat, nasal congestion, coughs, and fever.

GOLDENSEAL ROOT/OREGON GRAPE ROOT POWDER: Since goldenseal is on the brink of extinction Oregon grape root may be substituted. Both have the same medicinal properties, but Oregon grape root is not as strong, so you have to use more of it. Internally either may be used as a natural antibiotic in the form of an infusion or in capsules. The taste of both is strong and disagreeable to the average palate. Children prefer the capsules, and for those too young to swallow capsules, mix the powder with olive oil and apply to bottoms of warmed feet. Used in the treatment of colds, flu, and inflammation. Externally used as a poultice for conjunctivitis and inflammation and as an ointment for wounds, rashes, and other skin irritations.

LAVENDER FLOWERS: Externally used as an infusion in the bath, as a calmative, relaxant, and sedative, and for headache.

PEPPERMINT LEAVES: Internally the leaves, as an infusion, or the oil is used for irritable bowel, colic, stomach cramps, vomiting, nausea, poor digestion, nervousness, and insomnia. Externally used as an infusion in the bath for itching skin conditions and as a steam bath for sinus congestion.

PLANTAIN LEAVES: Externally used as a decoction for bites, stings, and ringworm.

SLIPPERY ELM POWDER: Internally used in the form of an infusion, or the raw powder is mixed with food or beverage, for inflammatory irritation, such as sore throat, and for diarrhea or constipation.

HERBAL TINCTURES

CALENDULA: Externally used for all open wounds and skin rashes. Internally used as a mouthwash for any kind of mouth sores.

CHAMOMILE: Used internally for digestive disturbances, nervousness and sleeplessness.

ECHINACEA: Internally used for the prevention and in early stages of colds, flu, sore throat, fever, earache, and inflammation.

PEPPERMINT: Used internally for colic, tummy aches and flatulence.

HOMEOPATHIC REMEDIES

The practice of homeopathy is based on an observation called *the law of similars.* In simple terms, this means that what a substance can cause, it can also cure. A substance can be used as medicine when symptoms that the patient is experiencing are similar to the symptoms that a healthy individual would experience if they were taking that same substance. There are many examples of the principle *like cures like.* Everyone knows how coffee keeps people awake and alert. In homeopathy coffee is used in dilution to cure patients with just the same kind of insomnia associated with an overly active mind. To find out more about how homeopathy works, refer to *Homeopathy: Beyond Flat Earth Medicine* by Timothy Dooley, N.D., M.D.

You will notice that I have relied heavily on the use of homeopathic remedies in this manual. This form of treatment may be unfamiliar to you, yet I encourage its use in the home. Homeopathic remedies are safe, easy to use, inexpensive, and have virtually no side effects. I feel it is well worth the effort to learn about this wonderful medicine.

When giving homeopathic remedies, pour out three pills at a time in the cap of the container, and place the pills in the child's mouth, preferably under the tongue. These little pills dissolve quickly, are pleasant to the taste, and are not meant to be chewed. I never met a child who didn't like taking them. If you are using the liquid form, half a dropperfull is one dose.

For general acute conditions, use homeopathic remedies in the 30c potency. Remedies are best absorbed when placed under the tongue. They are, however, still effective when simply placed in the mouth.

Note: *Homeopathic remedies do not work as well if camphor has been rubbed on the skin. Do not ingest mint or caffeine when taking remedies as these substances may antidote or diminish the properties of homeopathics.*

KEEP THE FOLLOWING HOMEOPATHIC REMEDIES IN YOUR HOME FIRST-AID KIT:

Aconitum napellus ~ Aconite: Indicated in the early sudden onset of many childhood diseases, including sore throat, earache, fever, croup, coughs, and colds. A child needing Aconite is usually anxious, restless, and fearful.

Allium cepa: Indicated for common cold symptoms, including watery nasal discharge, watery eyes, and reddened, irritated eyes, nostrils, and upper lip.

Apis mellifica ~ Apis: Indicated for bites and stings where there is much swelling with burning, stinging pains, and for other itchy, red, swollen skin irritations.

Arnica montana ~ Arnica: Indicated for all bumps, bruises, strains, and sprains, and for head injuries, eye injuries, shock, and pain from physical labor.

Arsenicum album ~ Arsenicum: Indicated for the anxious, restless child suffering from burning pains in the head, stomach, or throat, or from chickenpox, sleeplessness, or sinus congestion.

Belladonna: Indicated for conditions with flushed, red, hot skin as with a high, radiating fever; sore throat and earache; glassy eyes; dilated pupils; hot head with cold extremities; and a dry mouth, tongue, throat, and nose.

Chamomilla: Indicated for the irritable, temperamental, sometimes angry child experiencing sleeplessness, teething, pain, indigestion, earache, diarrhea, or asthma.

Gelsemium: Indicated for the mentally and physically weak child experiencing a headache, anxiety, influenza, or the measles.

Hepar sulphuricum ~ Hepar sulphur: Indicated for the touchy, irritable, quarrelsome, impatient child suffering from colds, coughs, croup, sore throats, or ear infections that are aggravated by a cold, chilly environment.

Hypericum: Primarily indicated for injuries to nerves or parts of the body rich with nerves. Especially helpful when the injury produces shooting pains or numbness. In addition to nerve injuries, it is useful for treating puncture wounds and animal bites.

Ipecacuahna ~ Ipecac: Indicated for nausea, vomiting, diarrhea, indigestion, nose bleeds, and headaches in the child who is hard to please, irritable, and impatient, who screams and yells until he gets what he wants, and then no longer wants it. Noise and especially music irritate this child.

Ledum palustre ~ Ledum: Indicated for puncture wounds, black eyes, bites, and stings, sprained ankles, and for pain relieved by cold applications.

Nux vomica: Indicated for the modern-day child who is physically and psychologically chilly and suffers from overindulgence in rich foods, junk food, alcohol, or drugs. It is also helpful to the hyperactive, overexcitable, irritable, rebellious child and for the child suffering from asthma, colic, hives, indigestion, insomnia, or nervous restlessness.

Oscillococcinum: A combination formula used for all symptoms associated with influenza. Its effects are especially beneficial when taken at the first sign of flu symptoms, including headache, body aches and pains accompanied by weakness and fever.

Pulsatilla: Indicated for the emotionally moody, sensitive child who craves sympathy and always feels better outdoors and suffers from asthma, bedwetting, conjunctivitis, common cold, earache, fever, mumps, measles, insomnia, sinusitis, headaches, or grief.

Rescue Remedy: Indicated for shock, hypertension, and anxiety. Produces a positive, calming, stabilizing effect in a wide range of stressful situations.

Rhus toxicodendron ~ Rhus tox: Indicated when symptoms are relieved by continuous motion and aggravated when suffering from poison oak or ivy, hives, chickenpox, backache, sprain, or strain.

Ruta gravelolens: Indicated for injuries to the knee, shin, ankle, or elbow, for sprains, especially when the injury feels hot to the touch, and for bruises that heal slowly. It is the most common remedy for tennis elbow or chronic knee injuries.

Silica : Indicated for the treatment of splinters.

Symphytum: Indicated for fractured bones, injuries to the soft tissue surrounding bones, and for sprained ankles, and very effective for injuries from being hit with a blunt instrument which does not break the skin and creates black and blue bruises, such as a black eye.

Urtica urens: Indicated for insect bites, stings, and burns.

SUPPLEMENTS

KEEP THE FOLLOWING SUPPLEMENTS ON HAND – LIQUID FORM IS EASIEST TO ADMINISTER TO BABIES AND SMALL CHILDREN:

Vitamin A

Vitamin C

Vitamin E

Combination of vitamin C with Echinacea

Garlic capsules

Zinc lozenges

Charcoal tablets

When it is not easy for babies and children to swallow tablets or capsules, give them liquid forms of herbs and supplements or rub the herbs on the bottoms of their feet as described earlier, under *Herbs in Bulk.*

You may have noticed that aspirin has not been suggested as part of a child's medicinary. *It is **never** recommended to give aspirin to anyone under the age of 20, because it has been known to cause Reye's Syndrome, which can be fatal to children and teenagers.*

Infant Care

BREAST FEEDING

Nursing your baby is the first contribution you make to ensure your child has a healthy body. Mother's milk provides perfect nutrition and antibodies important to ward off infection. Aside from the nutritional benefits, great emotional needs are met when nursing your baby, for both the mother and infant.

If you are unable to nurse your child, goat's milk is a good supplement to the infant diet. It should not be used exclusively, however, because it has too much sodium and not enough sugar. It is closest to mother's milk in its nutritional make-up. Very few babies are allergic to goat's milk the way many are to cow's milk or soy formulas.

Introduce your infant to a bottle as early as possible, even if you have chosen to breast feed. Express breast milk and keep it in the freezer until ready to use, or rely on one of the other alternatives mentioned. Occasional feedings by other loved ones will give you a little freedom, and get baby used to feeling comfortable in the care of others. When this practice is introduced early, it makes for a much less traumatic transition later, so that both mother's and child's needs are met, and everyone can feel happy and secure. If you are not breast feeding, remember to hold your child in your arms when giving her a bottle. Your breath, your heartbeat, the feel of your skin and the eye contact are vital ways in which you transmit health and well-being to your baby.

Avoid the modern day practice of propping up a bottle on a pillow and leaving your child alone during feedings. Infancy is a very short period of life and a crucial stage of development, when baby needs a lot of contact with mother to ensure successful emotional development as well as the meeting of physical needs.

Babies, like animals, equate food with love. Regular cuddling also helps the mother stay connected and in touch with the baby's desires. The more you hold your child, the more you will be able to intuit when something is wrong or right!

MASTITIS

It is not uncommon for mothers to develop mastitis, a breast infection, which is detectable by a painful, hot, red area on the breast caused by plugged milk ducts. This usually occurs when you've gone a little longer than usual between feedings. I had a couple of episodes myself and found a simple solution that worked every time. First try a hot wash cloth, as hot as you can tolerate, placed directly on the inflamed area for about three to five minutes. Then put baby on the breast to feed. As the milk begins to let down, place four fingers flat on your breast, and massage down toward the nipple. The heat and gentle pressure should unblock the duct and encourage the milk to flow. If this isn't effective alone, shred a fresh **raw beet** and place this poultice on the breast between feedings. It feels good and should do the trick. If neither of these remedies works, consult your healthcare practitioner. Supplement your immune system at this time with **Echinacea, goldenseal** and **vitamin C.** This is also a time when more rest is advisable.

SWADDLING

As your baby develops inside the womb, he is kept warm, secure, protected, and confined. Swaddling is a way to duplicate a womb-like environment for your baby after he is born. Start by rubbing in the *vernix caseosa*, the white creamy substance that coats your newborn's skin at birth, instead of washing it off. This is nature's protective coating, which keeps baby's skin soft and smooth. Hold off on the full-body bath for a few days if possible. Of course, you'll need to keep the bottom washed and the face wiped clean. Once you start to bathe your baby, make sure to hold him very securely while he's in the water. It's best if you can get in the tub yourself and hold him against your torso. Use soft little towels to dry him and keep him covered as much as possible. Dress baby in loose-fitting clothes, then swaddle him.

Swaddling is the art of wrapping your child in such a way that the arms and legs are not left flailing, and the neck is not left unsupported. Simulate the warmth and security of the womb. Take a cotton receiving blanket and lay your baby's head in one corner of it. Fold up the bottom triangle of the blanket, so that it covers the torso, and then fold over each side, one at a time. You can wrap the blanket just under his armpits, so baby is free to move his hands and arms. Now your child is in a nice secure bundle, easy for you to hold and carry. If it's hot outside, still bundle loosely in a light cotton or rayon receiving blanket, after dressing him in a T-shirt and diaper only. A swaddled baby feels safe and secure in the overwhelming world outside the womb.

IMMUNIZATION

Immunization is a controversial subject for those leaning towards natural healthcare. After extensive research and soul-searching and with the avid support and recommendation of Dr. Bernard Jensen, D.C., I decided not to vaccinate my children with the exception of tetanus. The reason I decided to give this one is because gardening is a lifestyle for me, and I always kept a pile of manure in the yard. I personally felt I would be doing more harm than good by giving all the recommended shots.

It is my belief that vaccinations greatly compromise the immune system and weaken a person's ability to fight infectious disease. This is plainly seen amongst adults who were blanketly immunized through the school system during the 1950s. This segment of our population is rampant with immune-deficient diseases, such as cancer, AIDS, chronic fatigue, fibromyalgia and lupus. The conscious choice not to vaccinate requires a sincere commitment. Education is essential. I learned to use homeopathic immunization in the form of *nosodes* (the potentized homeopathic remedies prepared from diseased tissue or the product of disease). They can be used to prevent or treat the associated disease. I took extra effort to feed my children high quality food, and to support their immune systems with vitamins, minerals, and herbs. There are many books that cover the reasons for and against vaccinations and also describe what is in them. I have listed several of these books so you can decide for yourself what would be best for your child:

The Immunization Decision by Randall Neustaeder, North Atlantic Press.
Immunization Theory vs. Reality by Neil Miller, New Atlantean Publications.
Vaccines: Are They Really Safe and Effective? by Neil Miller, New Atlantean Publications.
Vaccination and Immunization: Dangers, Delusions, and Alternatives by Leon Chaitow, C.W. Daniel.
Homeopathy and Immunization by Leslie Speigh, C.W. Daniel.

Part 2

CONDITIONS

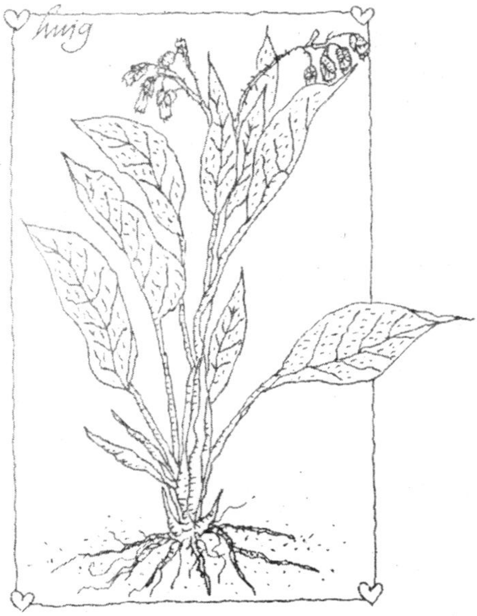

It is always wise to consult the naturopathic physician of your choice for a diagnosis when you attempt to treat your child. After you have the diagnosis, and you know what it is you are treating, then you and your practitioner can discuss how you will actually treat your child. Your knowledge in coming up with a treatment plan is very important. Don't be afraid to get involved. As you develop a relationship with your physician, you will find that he or she will encourage your healthcare education and be very supportive.

Acne

In addition to the physical aspect, acne carries with it a huge and sometimes overwhelming psychological burden. It's embarrassing, unattractive, worrisome, and painful. Over-the-counter treatments can get expensive, and most of them don't help much. Pharmaceuticals are even more costly, and they all have side effects, such as yeast infections; red, dry, burning, itchy, flaky skin; and an intolerance to sunlight. During acne-prone years, oils are present on the teenager's skin that decrease during the rest of one's life. Special care of the skin is necessary during this period. Provide your child with a gentle, cleansing face wash using **Calendula, Aloe vera,** or **lavender** in the ingredients. There are many fine products on the market for this purpose. Your child needs a gentle voice, reassuring words, genuine compliments, and encouragement during this uncomfortable time.

Diet plays a major role in managing acne. Avoid dairy products, especially if the blemishes are concentrated around the hairline. Reduce greasy, oily, and fast foods. Give your child plenty of fresh fruits and vegetables, purified water, and regular exercise. The best treatment we found was a botanical combination of **burdock, yellow dock, and dandelion root** in the form of a tincture. My youngest son had to deal with the unfortunate experience of acne. It's hereditary in our family, and at first nothing helped. Good diet, exercise, face washes, and topical creams just didn't make the difference we were looking for. My oldest child was working for a local naturopathic pharmaceutical company at the time, and she suggested the above formula. He took the remedy faithfully, 15 drops of the tincture in a glass of juice or water twice a day. After two months he was a handsome sight to behold. These herbs are well known for liver detoxification and blood purification. By using this natural remedy, he cleared up his complexion, cleansed his liver, revitalized the blood stream, and suffered zero side effects.

Asthma

Asthma occurs when the airways in the lungs become blocked to the passage of air. The symptoms of asthma include breathing which gradually becomes labored and a wheezing sound, which is heard with each breath. If you look carefully at the child's chest as she breaths, you will notice that her skin seems as though it sticks to the ribs when she takes air into the lungs. This condition gradually becomes worse over a few hours. She struggles for breath and becomes fearful, anxious, nervous, and tense. Asthma can be a serious and possibly life-threatening condition. Children and babies with asthma should receive medical attention. Keep in mind that conventional drugs used for asthma can impair immune function and cause side effects that can lead to more serious health problems.

There are a variety of possible causes related to asthma attack. Weak lungs due to hereditary factors, tuberculosis, and repeated lung infections are primary causes. Emotional factors are very important to notice in children over three years old. The emotional factors that are likely to cause stiffening of the muscles in the chest are unexpressed anger, tension, and fear related to stress in the family. It is not uncommon to see children with asthma when the parents do not get along or are getting a divorce. Asthma can also occur when a child experiences a parent as dominant or overcritical. She may feel as though she hasn't room to breathe. Asthma attacks are often triggered by allergies to food, house mites, dust, animal hair, molds, artificial colorings and flavorings, and pollen.

Asthma, continued

No matter what the cause, there are some treatments that can give your child some relief during asthma attacks. Homeopathic **Aconite 30c** is very useful at the first sign of asthmatic breathing, especially if anxiety and fear are present. **Arsenicum 30c** should be considered if the child is restless, and if, as the asthma attack continues, the child becomes more and more fearful and you notice that she can breath better when sitting up erect. **Chamomilla 30c** should be used if the asthma attack is brought on by a tantrum. It is also indicated when a child has a hard, dry cough and when being in cold air or drinking cold water relieves her breathing.

Comfrey ointment can be massaged into the chest for about five minutes. This is a soothing, relaxing, and tension-relieving treatment. Avoid mucus-producing foods, especially milk and cheese, during asthma attacks. Concentrate on easily digested foods, such as steamed rice and vegetables, soups, and herbal teas, such as **chamomile tea.** Gentle exercise such as walking encourages fresh air in the lungs and also strengthens the immune system. Take her for a walk in a park where there are ducks to feed or pleasant flowers to smell and discover. Vigorous exercise should be avoided as it may cause wheezing and bring on an asthma attack. Plenty of sleep is essential in healing any illness. The body's tissues are restored and deep-seated diseases are cured during sound, restful sleep. Read your child a story and encourage her to nap. Lie beside her until she falls asleep if there is any indication of fear associated with her asthma attacks. This will reassure her that all is well in the world and she can relax and breathe freely.

Attention Deficit Disorder and Hyper-activity

According to statistics, this frequently over- or mis-diagnosed modern day condition is on the rise. Are all these children really suffering from an illness? Or are they merely displaying a temperament that society is becoming less tolerant of? Before you label your child, ask yourself this question: are there really more kids with ADD or has our tolerance for active behavior decreased?

I believe many are highly intelligent, mentally active, bright, healthy children who require a different learning style than what is forced on them in our schools. They process information so fast that they easily become bored in an ordinary classroom where they are expected to adopt a routine that is impossible for children of their temperament. These are special kids with special needs. Society calls them hyperactive. They are quick minded, eager to learn, love to figure things out, and have to keep moving. They need encouragement, acknowledgement, and praise. In the ordinary classroom they are bored, disruptive, and intolerable because they are confined in what they consider an intolerable situation.

My oldest son displays the hyperactive personality. He was the kind of kid who could never get enough attention and was always making us laugh or scream at the dinner table. He was fussy, irritable, and hard to please. Sound familiar? These kids require more stimuli than the average child. They love a challenge and need to keep busy or they disrupt the family, the classroom, and the community. Many of these kids grow up to be criminals because their behavior has been improperly channeled. If your child is spinning his wheels and can't sit still and is driving you crazy, ride the horse in the direction it's going. Give hyperactive kids hyper-activity, both mental and physical. Don't try to sedate and force them to sit still.

One of my favorite ways to play with my son when he seemed too full of energy was to present him with a

Attention Deficit Disorder, continued

challenge. This temperament loves competition. I would start by asking him a question. 'How long do you think it will take you to run around the block?' He'd say sixty seconds and, of course, I'd challenge him by saying I didn't think he could run that fast. So he would run off to prove me wrong as I started to count one, two, three, and so on until he came back. Well, of course, he'd have to run around a few more times trying to beat his record until he was exhausted and ready to sit down for awhile. This was a great solution to hyperactivity just before lunch. Then we could all sit down to eat without the usual fuss we'd normally have to put up with at mealtimes. By choosing this sort of activity you will not only calm your child down, but you'll also create a situation that will result in positive acknowledgement instead of punishment. Don't forget to reward your child whenever possible. Go out of your way to set him up to succeed.

These children love to figure things out and they are good at it. Many hyperactive kids love numbers and math. Have your child count all the coins in the money jar, stack them up neatly and then let him know how smart he is and what a big help he has been. Now reward him with some of the coins and ask him to figure out what he started with and what is left after he subtracts his reward. Have him divide up all his blocks or cars by size or color, categorize them, count them, divide them, and make it a game to challenge his thinking. The whole family will be happier when this child's behavior is channeled into positive activity and encouraged instead of oppressed.

There are proven links between diet and behavior. Help your child by eliminating toxic substances, such as artificial flavorings, colorings, and preservatives. Some children are affected by even minute traces of pesticides, herbicides, and chemical fertilizers. Organic food can make a dramatic difference to these hypersensitive children. Check your child for food allergies. Begin by eliminating milk, peanuts, and oranges. Remember to give

Attention Deficit Disorder, continued

your child purified water to drink every day. Encourage him to begin the day with a glass of purified water to get things going properly and to help flush out toxins. Give him water to drink when he is thirsty, instead of juice, pop or other artificial, chemical-laden beverages. Try some of the fruit flavored teas on the market, such as strawberry-kiwi, which makes a pleasant tasting, visually pleasing beverage for kids. Add some lemon, lime, or orange slices.

Treating your child for ADD and hyperactivity with homeopathy will require a visit to a naturopathic physician or a homeopathic practitioner. It is necessary to document all the particulars of your child's behavior to determine which remedy would be most helpful. The constitution of the child has to be analyzed and there might be some trial and error involved before arriving at the desired remedy. A little patience in this process will be well worth the effort.

To find out more about natural treatments for ADD and hyperactivity read *Natural Treatments for ADD and Hyperactivity* by Skye Weintraub, N.D., and *Ritalin Free Kids* by Judyth Reichenberg-Ullman, N.D. and Robert Ullman, N.D.

Bites and Stings

You can prevent mosquito bites by using any natural repellent that contains **citronella oil.** Apply as directed on the container whenever your child will be exposed to mosquitoes. Once a bite occurs, swab **white** or **apple cider vinegar** on the welt. This will stop the itch and reduce the swelling.

Use homeopathic **Ledum 30c** for any puncture wound, including bites and stings. Give three tablets as soon as you notice a bite or sting. Spider bites should be suspected whenever you or your child has an itchy, red, and possibly painful bite and no idea how or when it happened. Give Ledum right away and then consider the following topical

Bites and Stings, continued

treatment. If you have some **plantain** growing in your yard (usually you will unless you have a chemical yard) pick two or three leaves, chew them up into a soft little wad, and place directly on the bite. Put a band-aid over it to hold the plantain in place and remove the band-aid when the plantain starts to dry out. If the bite or sting produces sharp shooting pains, give **Hypericum 30c.**

Wasp, hornet, and bee stings hurt a lot and frighten children. First give **Rescue Remedy** to calm your child down. Give half a dropperfull in the liquid form, or place three pills on or, preferably, under the tongue. Prepare a **baking soda compress** by mixing baking soda and cool water to form a paste, and apply this directly on the sting. Brush off the paste when it's dry. If you haven't any baking soda, make a **mud compress** by mixing water and soil to make the paste, and apply this directly to the sting.

There are two homeopathics to keep on hand specifically for bee stings. **Ledum 30c**, previously mentioned, and **Apis mellifica 30c**. Try Ledum first, and if results are not obvious within 15 minutes, give a dose of Apis mellifica. Both of these remedies relieve the pain and swelling associated with bites and stings. Apis also relieves the itching that develops a few hours to one day later. If the reaction to the bee sting is severe, such as abnormal swelling, signs of shock, or difficulty breathing, call emergency services immediately.

Bumps, Bruises, and Sprains

Children fall down a lot, banging their little heads, especially when they start walking. **Arnica 30c** is always good for these small injuries, and just as good for really serious ones as well. Always keep some around the house and in your purse or car. It will come in handy at sports games and on your trips to the park. **Arnica oil or ointment** can be used topically on sprains, bumps, and bruises as long as the skin is not broken. If the skin is broken, resort to **Calendula succus** (Calendula in an

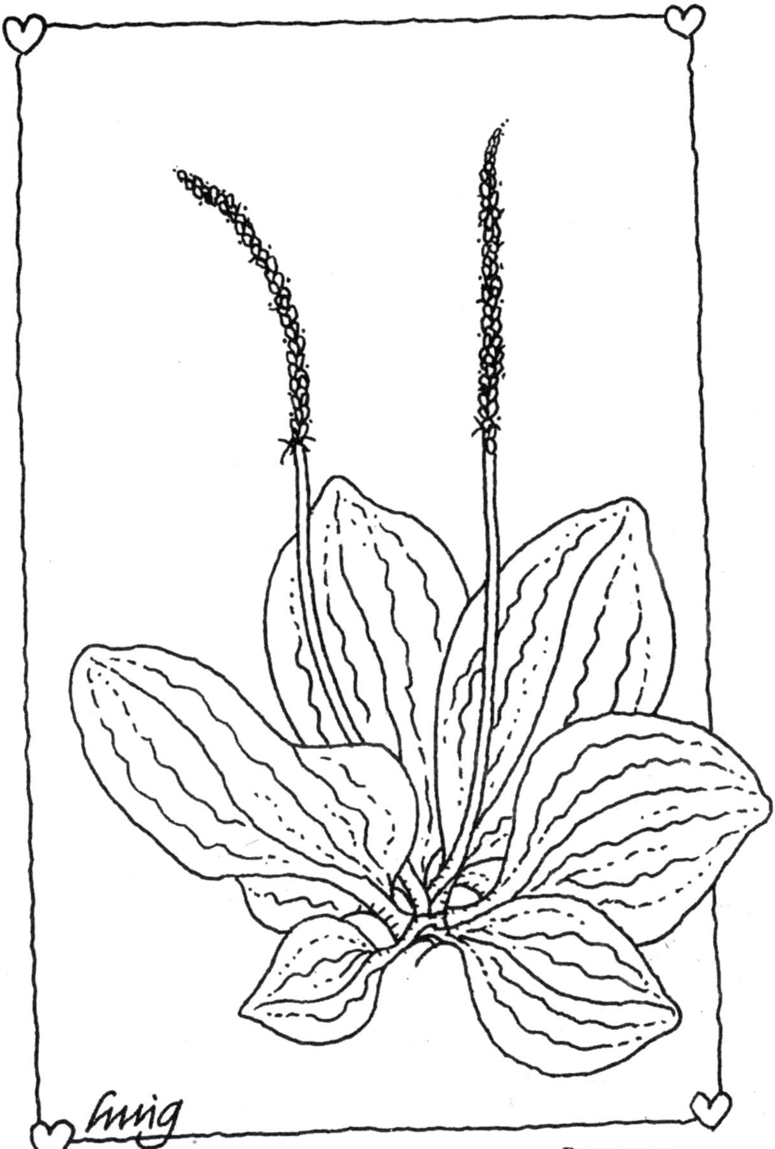

PLANTAIN

Bumps, Bruises and Sprains, continued

alcohol base) or **ointment. Calendula tea** swabbed on open wounds will heal them quickly, and never burns or causes pus. **Ledum 30c** is used if the injury turns black and blue, especially if the injury is caused by a blow from an object and feels cool to the touch. Alternate Ledum 30c and Arnica 30c for a black eye and wounds that are sensitive to touch. If the wound is warm, use **Hypericum 30c** along with the Arnica. Hypericum 30c is used when there is some damage to nerves.

Apply ice, ice packs, or a cold wash cloth on swollen or red bruises. When the ankle or foot is involved, elevate the leg during cold applications.

Make a **comfrey compress** for really bad bruises by steeping a handful of fresh or dried comfrey leaves in a quart of hot water for five to ten minutes. Do not boil them. After steeping, remove the leaves and place them inside a thin cotton sock or piece of muslin. Comfrey has prickly leaves, so make sure you do not put the plant directly on the bruise. (This could cause minor contact dermatitis.) Dip your compress in the remaining tea, squeeze slightly, and place directly on the bruise. Using bandage tape or a strip of cloth, fasten the compress to the body. Let your child sleep with the compress on the bruise over night. You'll be amazed in the morning to see that the bruise will be significantly lighter and less tender than the night before.

Burns

For minor burns, give the remedy **Urtica urens 30c** right away. You'll know the remedy is working because the child will cease to cry or complain. When the remedy wears off and complaining resumes, give the remedy again.

Minor burns can be treated topically with **baking soda** mixed with cool water to form a soft paste, which you apply directly to the burn. This is both soothing and cooling and will prevent scarring. You can also swab **Aloe vera gel** on the wound. You can use store-bought gel, or if you have an

Burns, continued

Aloe vera plant that is three years or older, you can use the plant itself. Cut a leaf at the base of the plant and peel off the outer skin to expose the gel-like substance and swab the burn generously with it several times a day. Store the remaining leaf in a plastic bag, and refrigerate until you want to reuse it. If you haven't any remedies on hand, soak the burn in cold water to relieve the pain.

Canker Sores

Too much acidity and poor digestion contribute to the formation of canker sores. Homeopathic **Borax 30c** given three times a day for a couple of days can help if your child suffers from canker sores. **Gentian violet** in liquid form works well, and usually brings relief. However, it can be very messy and leaves a temporary stain on whatever it touches. **Calendula tea** as a mouthwash is also effective. Keep the diet alkaline by staying away from sweets and acid juices, such as orange and tomato juice. Yogurt with acidophilus feels cool to the mouth and promotes good digestion.

Chickenpox

All my children got the chickenpox, one right after the other. Usually the older the child, the more uncomfortable she is. Most children feel well enough to play indoors, but keep them out of school and away from other children because chickenpox is very contagious.

Keep the patient as cool as possible. Cool rooms, cool water, and cool drinks are beneficial. **Calendula tea** swabbed on the scabs helps stop the burning itch that most children experience. Make Calendula tea by pouring a cup of boiling water over a tablespoon of dried flowers. Let the tea steep for five to ten minutes, and then place in the refrigerator to cool. Swab the cooled tea on the scabs that really itch.

Two homeopathic remedies are particularly good to try at the very onset of chickenpox: **Aconite 30c** or **Arsenicum**

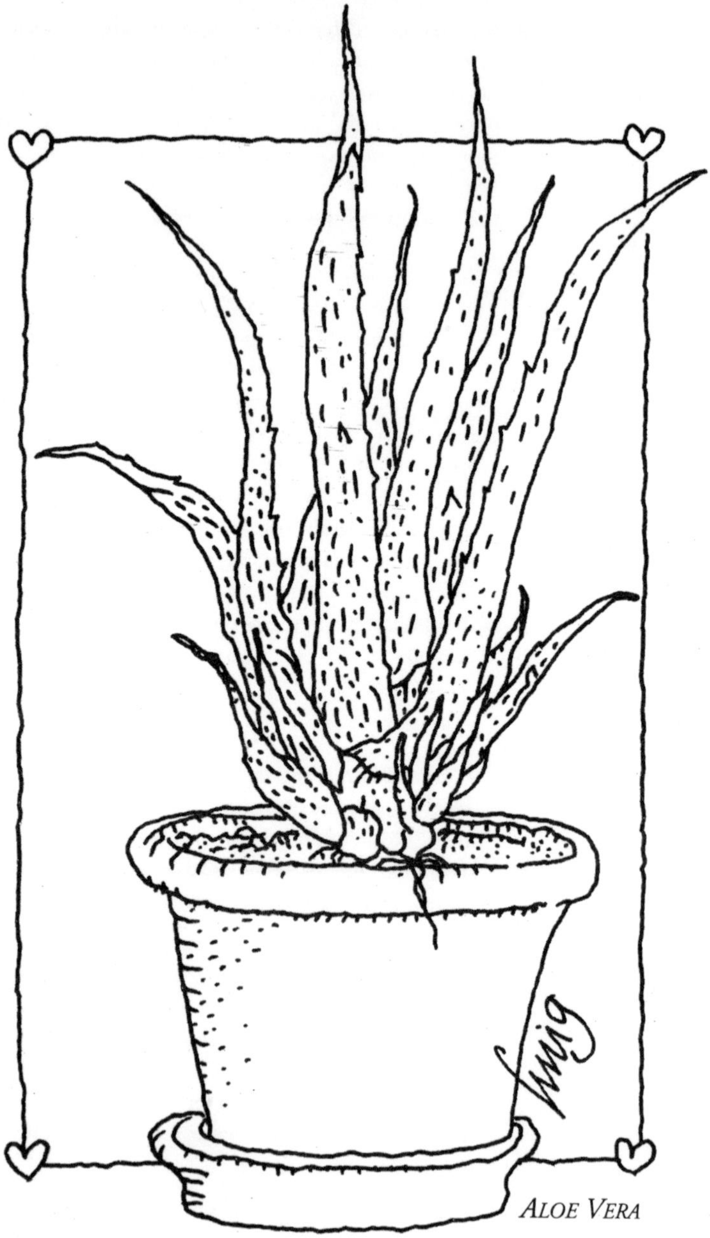

ALOE VERA

Chickenpox, continued

30c. In my family I was the first to show signs, with the little blisters appearing on my neck and face. I took only one dose of Arsenicum 30c, and in a day or two all the blisters had completely disappeared. Unfortunately, my children were not so lucky. They all got full-blown chickenpox. My daughter, who was the oldest, suffered the most. The boys were fairly well covered with skin eruptions, but somehow it didn't seem to bother them much.

You can use the following remedies for the prevailing symptoms: **Rhus tox 30c** for severe, intense itching and restlessness in the night; **Apis mellifica 30c** for itchy, stinging eruptions that are worse with heat and better with cold; **Belladonna 30c** if the child appears sick and drowsy, with a headache or fever, flushed face, and is unable to sleep.

A tepid bath before bed can help with the discomfort. Remember to blot the skin dry rather than rubbing, which can add to the itchiness and possible scarring if you rub scabs off prematurely. Chickenpox is a very common childhood disease and shouldn't cause too much distress in young children. Teenagers will tend to be very uncomfortable. Try giving them **Arsenicum 30c** at the very first sign of blisters, and maybe they will be as lucky as I was. If at all possible, discourage your child from scratching off the scabs as this can cause scarring. If some scarring does occur, rub a little **vitamin E oil** on the scars after all the scabs are completely dried up.

Circumcision

Don't! Over half the male babies on the planet are not circumcised. Let nature take its course. Care of the uncircumcised penis is easy. Just keep it clean like you would the rest of the body. As for pulling back the foreskin, boys tend to do this on their own as soon as they can touch themselves. Until they start to do this, gently move the foreskin back as far as it will go, without forcing

Circumcision, continued

it, when you give him a bath. My boys got a few minor infections. This condition is easily relieved by gently pulling the foreskin back to the area of inflammation, and applying a small amount of **olive oil** with a Q-Tip or your finger tip, followed by a sprinkle of **goldenseal powder** on the red, swollen area. Release the foreskin back over the penis, and by the next day, things should be back to normal. If not, repeat one more day. A good time to apply this treatment is after an evening bath just before bedtime.

Colic

Colic is a problem that some babies are born with and tend to outgrow within three months. Signs of colic include diarrhea, nausea, vomiting, and restlessness, and frequently the infant feels very weak and sweaty. Slightly older children sometimes suffer from colic that is related to liver congestion. You can take some precautions to lessen the chance of your child getting colic or to reduce its severity. Encourage your baby to eat slowly and avoid agitation during feeding time. During the nursing years, mother should avoid the brassicas: the family of vegetables which includes cabbage, broccoli, and cauliflower. Other potential irritants are orange juice, lettuce, and rich and spicy foods. Give yourself time to relax when breastfeeding. If your baby is on cow's milk, try substituting goat's milk as it is much easier to digest. Avoid feeding your baby bananas, yogurt, or cold foods.

Two homeopathic remedies are especially helpful for colic. **Chamomilla 30c** is given to infants who are also teething. It is indicated for a baby who doubles up, kicks and screams, and has an abdomen that is sensitive to touch. Such a baby gets some relief from external heat, and by being carried with a gentle bouncing motion or by being rocked. **Nux vomica 30c** is useful when the baby wants to vomit or strains to defecate, but can't. These symptoms may develop in a breast-fed baby whose mother has eaten

Colic, continued

rich or spicy foods, drinks alcohol, or takes drugs. Try either one of these remedies at the onset of digestive irritability. Place three pills on or under your child's tongue or half a dropperfull in the liquid form. If the first remedy you try does not give relief within half an hour, try the other. Only one of my children had colic and he was greatly relieved with **peppermint oil**. Mix three drops of peppermint oil in two ounces of purified water and give a half a dropperfull to your baby when she is suffering from colic. The peppermint oil relaxes the stomach muscles and relieves the pain.

Massage is also helpful. Massage the baby's abdomen from the right to left side in a soft, yet firm, rotating motion before and after feeding. General back massage is comforting as well. Sometimes baby is more comfortable in an upright position, with her head on your shoulder, than she is lying flat on her back. A warm hot-water bottle or hot pack can be very comforting. Place the hot-water bottle on your lap or on your breast. Place a small, thin towel over the bottle and lay your baby on the towel, making sure that the baby's skin does not come in direct contact with the bottle, and that the bottle is warm, not hot. Burping the colicky baby is especially important.

Common Cold

Everybody, young and old alike, has to deal with a cold now and then. There are things you can do to lessen the discomfort, and as I've said before, early treatment can often prevent a mild symptom from developing into something more serious.

As soon as you detect a little sneeze, sniffle, or sore throat, think of the **wet sock treatment**. Begin with a warm foot bath. Always use the same temperature that you use when giving your child her regular bath. Soak her feet for at least eight minutes. Have ready a bowl of ice water in which you soak a pair of cotton socks. After the foot bath, dry off the feet and place the cold, wet, wrung-out socks on your

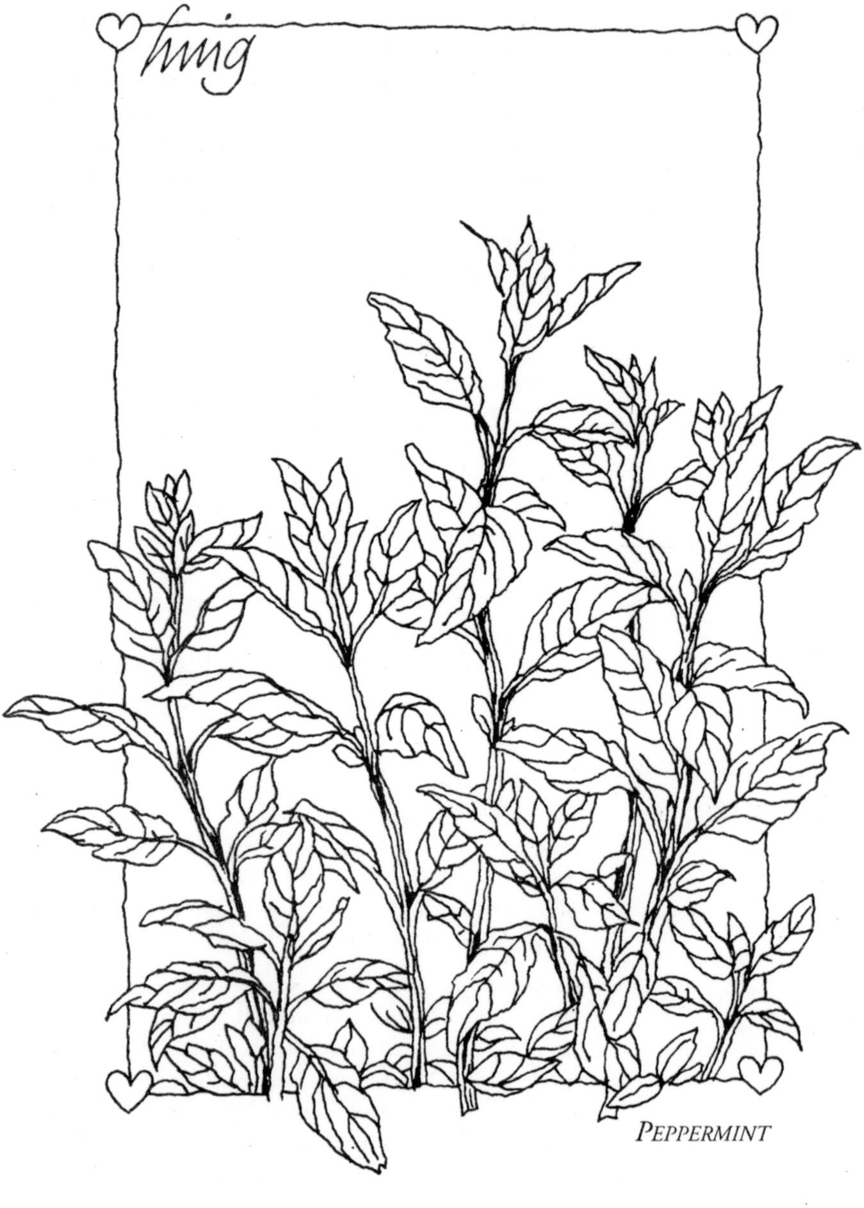

PEPPERMINT

Common Cold, continued

patient. Next place a pair of wool socks over the cotton socks. Wool is always preferred, but you can substitute polar fleece. Put your child in a nice warm bed, and by morning she should wake up smiling with the socks completely dry. This procedure stimulates the body's immune system and works well on patients of all ages. It's easy to do and doesn't cost any more than the price of a good pair of socks. Be sure to have some on hand so you'll be prepared.

No matter which symptoms occur first – sneezing, coughing, runny nose, sore throat, chills, or fever – begin by boosting the immune system with natural antibiotic herbs such as **Echinacea, garlic,** and **goldenseal.** None of these herbs are pleasant to the palate, so give them in capsules, taken with a full glass of water or in liquid form mixed with tea or juice. Follow the directions on the container for dosages. If you are treating a child too young to swallow these herbs in capsule form or one who refuses the liquid, prepare the herbs as follows:

Begin by giving your child a warm bath or foot bath to open the pores on the soles of her feet. Press one clove of garlic and mix with one-half teaspoon Echinacea powder, one-half teaspoon goldenseal powder, and one teaspoon of olive oil. Mix the combination in the palm of your hand and rub into the bottoms of her feet. Now put on a pair of cotton socks over the herbal mixture you have just rubbed in. This is a gentle way to administer herbs to your child. The warmth of the bath and the massaging with the oil mixture will sooth, relax, and nurture. Right before bed is the perfect time to apply this remedy.

Homeopathy is very beneficial for many of the symptoms frequently referred to as the common cold. **Allium cepa 30c** is indicated when excretions from the eyes and nose are clear and runny, and the eyes, nostrils, and upper lip are reddened and irritated. This remedy has also been effective for coughs associated with the previous symptoms. Place three pills under the tongue or give one half of a dropperfull at the first sign of cold symptoms.

Common Cold, continued

If the sinuses are plugged up and breathing is difficult after a child has experienced a chill, **Arsenicum 30c** brings relief.

You can find other remedies for colds by looking up the prevailing symptoms, such as sore throat, cough, fever, and sinus congestion in the table of contents of this book.

Conjunctivitis

Conjunctivitis is inflammation of the white part of the eye. The eye appears red and swollen, and possibly oozing. It is crusty after sleep and somewhat painful. Prepare **Calendula and goldenseal tea** by placing one cup of dried Calendula flowers and one teaspoon of goldenseal powder in a quart jar, and fill with boiling water. Let the tea steep about five minutes. Strain off the tea and place the herbs in a clean cotton sock or muslin bag. Soak this in the tea and apply directly to the closed eye. Do this while the tea is still warm; it feels very good. Swab the eye in this way with the tea several times throughout the day. The eye should look better in 24 hours. Repeat until all the symptoms are gone. Continue with internal supplements for immune support, such as **Echinacea, vitamins A and C,** and **garlic** for at least another week.

Constipation

Constipation is a problem caused by poor dietary habits, weak intestinal muscles, liver congestion, too much processed food, not enough water, and sometimes emotional distress. Begin by increasing the child's water intake with a glass of water first thing in the morning before any food is taken. Simplify the diet: minimize processed food and maximize steamed vegetables and soups. Gentle herbs for constipation are **Aloe vera** and **slippery elm.** Use Aloe vera in the liquid form and follow the instructions on the bottle. Slippery elm powder is known for its ability to

Constipation, continued

regulate the bowel. Mix a teaspoon of the herb in your child's applesauce or oatmeal. You can also mix a teaspoon of the powdered herb in a glass of water or juice and feed it to your child by the spoonful. Children usually do not object to its neutral taste. Foods that help relieve constipation include real maple syrup, figs, prunes or prune juice, and fresh pears. Herbal laxatives should be used with great care where babies and young children are concerned because of the danger of prolonged diarrhea. Seek the advice of a qualified practitioner under these circumstances.

Coughs

When treating a cough, first increase your child's liquid intake. Make sure she is drinking lots of water, and add teas to the diet. Boost the immune system when kids and babies get coughs and colds. For infants, mix **goldenseal and Echinacea powder** with some freshly ground **garlic.** Make a paste solution by mixing a combined teaspoon of these herbs in powdered form with a tablespoon of **olive oil.** After bathing your child, rub the mixture on the bottoms of her feet and put cotton socks on over the mixture. Rubbing herbal mixtures on the bottoms of the feet is a great way to give a fussy, uncooperative child herbal remedies. Older children can take these herbs in pill or liquid form.

Teas with **licorice** and/or **cherry bark** are specific for cough relief. They also taste good. Add a slice of lemon or orange to the tea. Give encapsulated Echinacea and goldenseal and increase vitamin C intake. These may also be given in liquid tincture form, but most tinctures are alcohol based and are unpleasant to the young palate. If you use tinctures, add a dropperfull to a cup of herb tea or a glass of water. They will barely detect the herbs. Give freely, three to four times per day. Put a vaporizer in the bedroom to keep some moisture in the air. Get some natural vapor balm that contains camphor and eucalyptus.

Coughs, continued

Rub the balm on the chest of children one year or older before bed, and also put the balm in the vaporizer. Excellent herbal cough syrups are available at local healthfood stores.

A great old-time remedy that works very well is the **hot onion poultice**. Take an ordinary yellow onion and slice and sauté it in olive oil until transparent. Let it cool off a bit. The onion should be placed directly on the upper chest, reaching up towards the throat. Apply while the onion is still very warm, as warm as the child can stand, and cover the onion with a washcloth or hand towel. (Check the temperature of the onion as you would check the temperature of a baby bottle on your wrist before application. Be very careful not to burn the skin and do not apply the onion mixture cold.) This substance may seem a little strange, but it actually feels very good. Your little one will love the soothing warmth. Make sure the child is warm and well covered. Remove the poultice once it has cooled, and rub the olive oil into the skin. It's important that your child is kept warm and gets a lot of rest when she has a cough. Keep a scarf or high-neck top around her throat when inside or outdoors, and make nap time a priority.

Coughs manifest in many different ways. Some come on suddenly. Some drag on for a long period of time. Some are productive with a discharge that is thin and watery or thick and gluey, or non-productive, where the cough is hard and dry, or wheezy and croupy with a tight feeling in the chest. There is also a feverish cough where the child is hot, weak, and experiences other discomfort. Make it your job to learn to describe and differentiate the coughs, so that you can consult a naturopathic practitioner and come up with a treatment that addresses the needs specific to your child's acute symptoms. If your child goes to bed feeling well, and wakes up with a dry, hoarse, croupy cough and his mouth is dry and he is very thirsty, **Aconite 30c** will give quick results. This remedy is also suggested for symptoms that come on suddenly and is commonly given for the initial stages for croup and bronchitis. For an

Coughs, continued

irritable child with a barking type cough, where you can hear mucus that cannot be coughed up rattling around in the chest, and where the child sweats while coughing, give **Hepar Sulpur 30c**.

You can purchase some very effective over-the-counter combination homeopathic remedies at health food stores and through the companies listed in the Directory. Look for remedies indicated for coughs, sore throat, fever, and so on. Keep these products on hand so you have something to give your little one at the very onset of symptoms. This is when homeopathy is most effective.

Cradle Cap

An easy, gentle treatment for cradle cap is to brush baby's head with a baby brush to loosen the flaky scalp, then rub a little **olive oil** on his head about an hour before bath time. When you bathe him, wash his head with baby shampoo, rinse, and towel dry. His condition should clear up in about three to five treatments, depending on the severity.

Cuts, Scrapes, and Minor Wounds

Children experience fear at the sight of blood. The way to alleviate this fear is to talk about the wound. Look your child straight in the eye and ask him how it happened, where it happened, and exactly what happened. He will calm down naturally as he speaks and explains his experience to you. Repeat whatever he says back to him in a gentle, soothing, caring tone. This process works very well with small children between the ages of two and seven.

When dealing with bleeding from cuts on the arms, hands, legs, or feet, raise the injured limb above the level of the heart to slow down and stop bleeding. If bleeding is profuse or you think stitches are required, call the

Cuts, Scrapes and Minor Wounds, continued

emergency room amd alert them that you are on the way and tell them the nature of the injury so that they will be ready for you when you arrive. To control the bleeding on the way, apply pressure over the wound with a sterile compress. *(Never apply pressure to head wounds.)* If the child is confused or upset, administer **Rescue Remedy** along with **Arnica 30c,** which may also be given for shock or stupor with shock. If the child is hysterical to the point of losing control, give him **Aconite 30c**.

Remember that a little blood can look like a lot to a child. Stay calm and your child will calm down.

Aconite 30c is the first homeopathic remedy to consider when your child experiences fear and anxiety with a minor wound. One dose should do the trick. If the fear and anxiety should return, give him another dose. **Arnica 30c** is given for the initial shock and trauma that a child experiences from injury. It is very effective for both internal and external bleeding. This is an essential remedy to keep in the car to be given to the victim of any automobile accident, whether it is minor or severe. An external application of **Calendula extract** or **tincture** reduces and stops bleeding and prevents infection. If you have Calendula growing in your yard, you can peel off the petals of one to three flowers, chew on them for a few seconds, and then apply them directly on the wound to stop bleeding. Calendula is easy to grow and a delightful addition to any garden.

Diaper Rash

So many people depend on convenience items, such as disposable diapers and disposable wash cloths. You may want to think twice about the impact of these items on the planet. A nice alternative to disposables is a diaper service. It costs about the same as disposables. The diapers are made of cotton instead of plastic, and they are reusable. Unfortunately, if you are using your own cloth diapers, your baby may be more prone to diaper rash. If you have this problem to contend with, the first solution is to give the bottom area as much air as possible. If you have some **mullein leaf** growing in your yard or a nearby vacant lot, cut a leaf off at the base and place it in the diaper so it covers the affected area. Once we were out camping and my daughter had quite a rash. We found some mullein leaf, placed it directly on the affected area overnight, and in the morning her diaper rash had disappeared. **Arrowroot powder** is also soothing, and it doesn't contain talc like so many expensive powders do. Talc has been proven to be carcinogenic.

A sitz bath in **Calendula tea** is also helpful for diaper rash. Make a strong tea with Calendula flowers (about a cup of flowers to a quart of water). Boil the water and pour over the flowers. Steep for eight minutes and pour the strained tea into a pot that is big enough for baby to sit and play in. Add enough cool water so the water level will be high enough to cover baby's entire bottom when she is placed in the bath. The temperature should be the same as her normal bath. Let her play in this solution for at least ten minutes. Sometimes mother's diet plays a role in diaper rash. If you are nursing and have been eating the brassicas, which include cabbage, broccoli, and cauliflower, avoid them. Orange juice has also been known to cause problems.

Diarrhea

Slippery elm powder will bring the bowel back into balance. For babies, mix a teaspoon of slippery elm powder in about a cup of water and feed it by the spoonful. An even easier method for a child old enough for solid food is to mix a spoonful of the powder in some applesauce or oatmeal and let the child eat it. Of course, homeopathy is the easiest medicine to use at any age. **Chamomilla 30c** is the first remedy to consider in simple cases of diarrhea, when bowel movements are greenish and bilious in character, or if signs of colic are present. One or two doses given about four hours apart is usually enough to bring about a change. Consider **Ipecacuanha 30c** if the diarrhea results from overeating and is accompanied by vomiting. **Charcoal tablets** can be used to bind things up if the child is old enough to swallow tablets (use two tablets at a time with a glass of purified water). For younger children, crush one and mix it in a glass of juice. Also correct the diet by feeding simple foods only. Rice with steamed vegetables is good. Add sweet potato to the diet and stay away from fruit juice and carbonated drinks. This is a good time to give a nice cup of herb tea to comfort and relax the child. **Chamomile tea** is a good choice.

Earache

All my children got earaches, but only one of them did so somewhat often and severely. My oldest boy suffered from intense, sharp, frightening pain. He would scream so loudly and frantically that he had me afraid he might be dying. Of course, he wasn't, and we were able to relieve him every time with homeopathy. First, I'd suggest getting the child off dairy products. Dairy products seem to consistently aggravate the condition. Increase his water intake. A gentle, soothing treatment for earaches is **mullein oil**. Begin by placing the bottle of mullein oil in a cup of hot water to warm it up a little. When it's warm, place three drops of the oil in the affected ear and massage the base of the ear to help the oil to drain down inside. Put

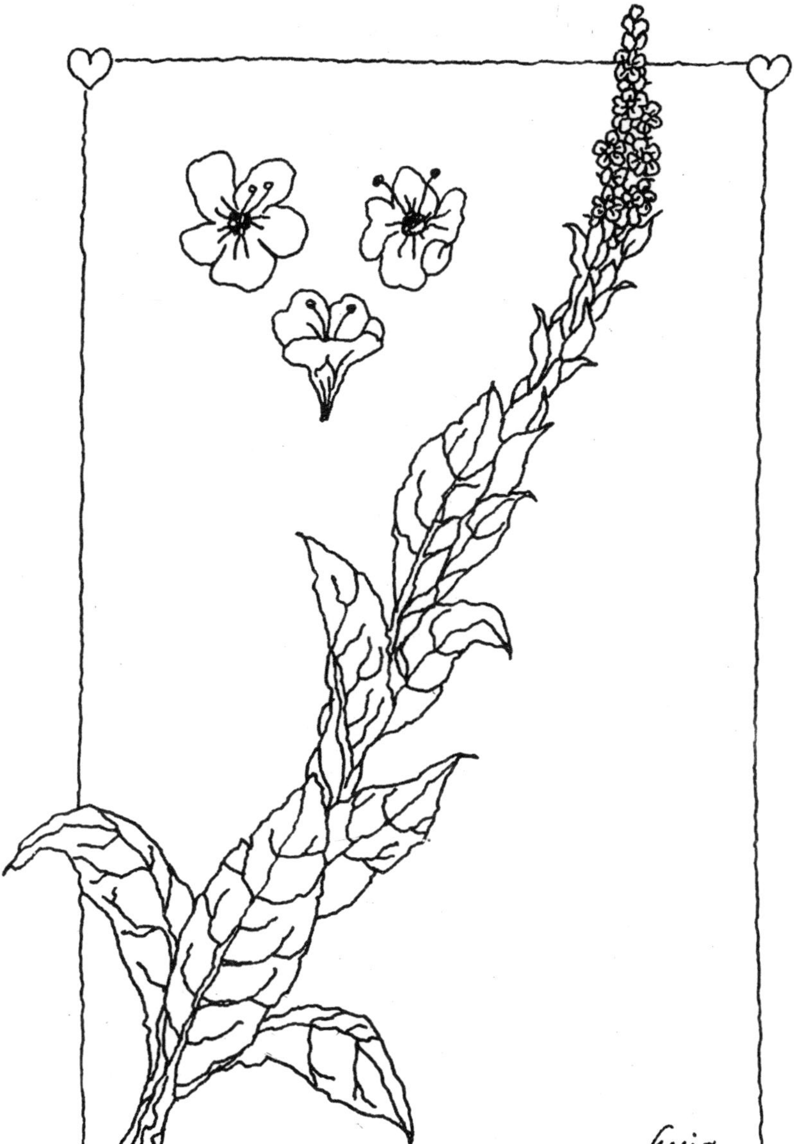

MULLEIN

Earache, continued

a little piece of cotton in the ear, put him to bed and give him a kiss goodnight. Caution: consult your physician before using eardrops to make certain that the eardrum is intact.

Several homeopathic remedies are indicated for earache. **Aconite 30c** is a good remedy when the earache comes on suddenly, especially after exposure to cold wind, or if your child experiences chills and fever after getting wet. If the child responds to the first dose and starts complaining again soon after, keep repeating the remedy every 15 minutes until the response holds. Frequently it took three to five doses before my son had constant relief. If the child stops complaining and says he has no more pain, then there is no need to repeat the remedy. If no relief comes after one or two doses over two to four hours, try a different remedy. **Belladonna 30c** is indicated if the child is glassy-eyed, red and hot, and delirious. Use **Chamomilla 30c** if your child has one hot red cheek, is cross, nervous, and hard to please. If the earache is mild and goes on for a long time, give **Pulsatilla 30c** three times a day for about three days.

A warm application is also comforting and relieves the pain. You can use a heating pad or, preferably, a hot water bottle or hot pack. Put a hand towel over the bottle or pack – do not place it directly on the skin. Over-the-counter combination remedies for sore throat and earaches, which do not require a prescription, are now readily available at health food stores or anywhere that sells natural medicines. About half a dropperfull or 3 pellets in the pill form is equivalent to one dose. A good indication that a remedy is working is if your child falls asleep soon after taking it. He will usually wake up feeling much better. This is a good time to rock the child, hold him close to your heart, and sing a little song.

JAMIE GOT THE MEASLES IN THE MONTH OF MAY

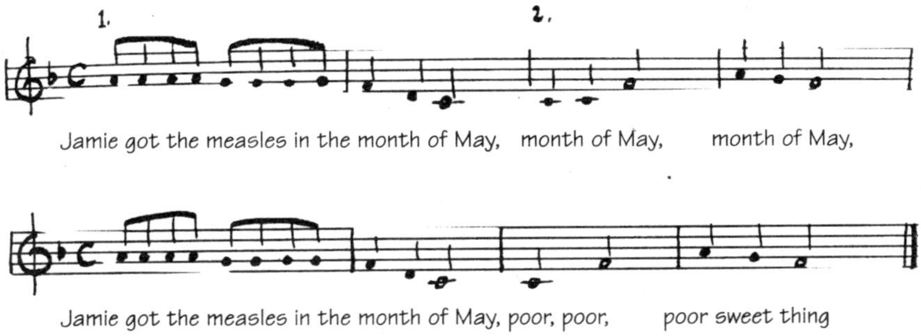

2. Mamma called the doctor with her pills and things, pills and things, pills and things,

   Mamma called the doctor with her pills and things, poor, poor, poor sweet thing.

3. Papa made some soup with a chicken wing, chicken wing, chicken wing,

   Papa made some soup with a chicken wing, poor, poor, poor sweet thing.

4. Nana made it better with a kiss and a hug, kiss and a hug, kiss and a hug,

   Nana made it better with a kiss and a hug, poor, poor, poor sweet thing.

5. Jamie got the measles in the month of May, month of May,

   Jamie got the measles in the month of May, poor, poor, poor sweet thing.

Fever

Feverish children can be a little scary. Remember that generally a fever means that your child has a healthy immune system, and that it's working properly in response to a deeper problem. Try to figure out what it is by noting other symptoms. Does she have a cough, sore throat, or stomach ache? Fever burns up the bugs. If the fever is fairly low (101°F or less), encourage the fever. Keep the patient warm, give her a bath, put her to bed in warm pajamas. Entice the body to sweat.

If the child has a higher fever, cool her down with a tepid sponge bath, and give her water to drink. Place a cool washcloth on her forehead. **Do not**, however, induce chills. Keep the patient in a warm room and under a blanket. Dehydration is often the biggest concern with fever, and water may not be enough. Give your child herb tea, diluted juices, or frozen juice bars.

For simple fever, one where no other symptoms are apparent, give **Aconite 30c** every two or three hours until perspiration starts, which indicates the body will soon cool down. If the child has a headache, is hot to the touch, red-cheeked, and glassy-eyed, give **Belladonna 30c.** If the fever doesn't yield readily to your treatment or if your child's temperature goes over 103°F a physician should be consulted.

Inflammation

Inflammation is often indicated by redness, swelling, and pain. If you suspect inflammation anywhere in the body, you can use the following treatment: pour a generous amount of **castor oil** on a clean washcloth or thick piece of flannel, place this directly on the inflamed area, and cover with a heating pad, hot water bottle or hot pack for 15 to 30 minutes. If you want to increase circulation in this area, alternate with an ice pack for 5 minutes. This treatment is used

Inflammation, continued

more frequently on adults, but can be used on a cooperative child. Because this treatment takes time, be prepared to read a long story or to watch a movie with your child while applying the castor oil compress.

In all cases of inflammation/infection, one should first boost the immune system. Give a combination of **Echinacea and vitamin C** immediately. This formula can be found in both liquid and pill form.

Garlic in capsule form can be given orally or the oil from the punctured capsule can be massaged into the bottom of the feet. This procedure works best if the feet have first been soaked in warm water. As usual, increase your child's water intake. If the inflammation is external (for example, if your boy has an infection on his penis and there is a red, swollen area) mix a little **goldenseal** powder with some olive oil. Gently push back the foreskin as far as is comfortable, and apply a little of the preparation to the inflamed area. One or two of these applications should stop the infection. This always worked for my boys.

Influenza

There is a very good commercial homeopathic remedy which works well when given at the onset of flu symptoms: **Oscillococcinum**. Remember this name and go buy some today so that you'll have it on hand when you need it. It comes with dosage instructions and it's very easy to use. If your child gets the flu, keep the diet light and simple, and increase steamed vegetables and soups. Give lots of water and herb teas. Homeopathic remedies for the flu include **Gelsemium 30c** for the very weak child who is content to lie still and has a mild fever with chills. **Belladonna 30c** is given when the pulse is small and rapid, the skin is hot and dry, the tongue is dry, and the child suffers from heat and pains in the head. **Baptisia 30c** is indicated when the child presents nausea and vomiting, a thickly-coated tongue, and possibly diarrhea.

Measles

None of my children got the measles. This contagious disease is characterized by cold symptoms, cough, irritation of the eyes, and high fever. A rash appears on the fourth day of the illness. There can be complications such as ear infections, pneumonia, and infection of the lymph nodes.

The suggested remedy for measles in Leslie Speight's book, *Homeopathy and Immunization* is the homeopathic prophylaxis **Morbillinum 30c**. This remedy can only be found through your naturopathic physician. Give three doses on the first day and then once a week until the trouble has passed. In Dana Ullman's book, *Homeopathy for Children and Infants,* he recommends **Aconite 30c** at the beginning stages of measles when the child has a high fever, a dry, barking cough, and reddened conjunctivas (pink eye) and when his skin burns and itches, and he feels restless, anxious, and frightened.

Belladonna 30c is often useful at the beginning stages of measles when there is sudden onset of high fever, a reddened face, and a throbbing headache. It is indicated when the child tends to be drowsy, a little delirious, and has difficulty falling and staying asleep, and when, despite the fever, he is not thirsty. **Gelsemium 30c** is indicated if the onset of symptoms are slow, if there is fever, weakness, and a sense of heaviness, both of the whole body and especially the eyelids, and if there is no thirst. Measles can be a serious disease. If you suspect measles, contact your pediatrician immediately.

Mumps

None of my children got the mumps. However, there was an outbreak of the disease while my boys were in grade school. A letter was sent home to all parents. I promptly gave my children the homeopathic prophylaxis **Parotidinum 30c**, which can only be obtained from your naturopathic physician. I gave three doses in one day. We had no occurrence of the disease.

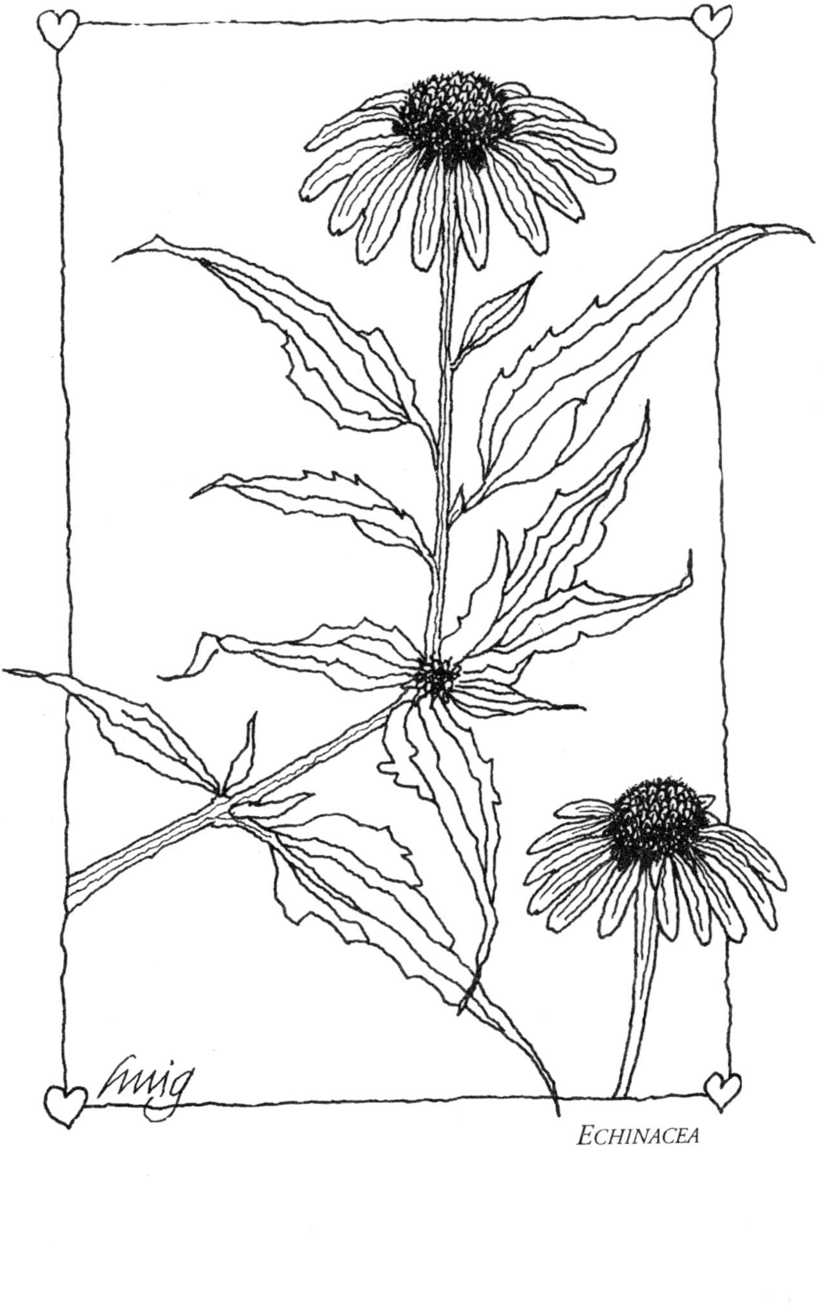

ECHINACEA

Mumps, continued

Mumps is highly contagious. It starts with a fever and the child has a headache and feels fatigued. Within 24 hours the child develops an ache near the lobe of the ear, and by the next day, the salivary glands in front of the ear become swollen. Pain occurs with chewing and on opening the mouth. The illness runs its course within six days. In Dana Ullman's book, *Homeopathy for Children and Infants* he recommends **Aconite 30c** at the beginning stages of mumps when the child has a sudden onset of fever, is restless, anxious, and very thirsty. **Belladonna 30c** is indicated if the child has a flushed face, and a throbbing headache and if he has swollen glands that are hot to touch and is drowsy but has difficulty sleeping.

If you suspect that your child is coming down with mumps, and especially if your teenager gets the mumps, contact your naturopathic physician immediately.

Nausea and Vomiting

The causes of nausea and vomiting vary, as do the antidotes. When your child suffers from motion sickness, whether it's due to traveling in a car, boat, or plane, give her **Cocculus 30c.** Cocculus works very well particularly if your child feels dizzy, nauseous, and is worse in the fresh air. Give **Tabaccum 30c** if your child child feels cold, faint, and sweaty, and feels some relief after vomiting.

Food poisoning is another story. Use **Arsenicum 30c** when your child has frequent bouts of offensive-smelling, burning diarrhea and feels nauseous with burning vomit. For Arsenicum to fit the picture, the child should complain that the diarrhea and vomiting burn. The child in an Arsenicum state is restless and anxious. Sips of warm water or **chamomile tea** will soothe her. Activated **charcoal tablets** greatly benefit children who are old enough to swallow the tablets. Charcoal tablets work quickly and should be used when you know the child has eaten something bad and is experiencing nausea,

Nausea and Vomiting, continued

vomiting, or diarrhea. Charcoal tablets are inexpensive and a great remedy to have on hand when traveling.

Ginger tea is good for tummy aches of any kind, and specifically those associated with nausea or vomiting. **Ginger ale** is also helpful and easily obtainable while you are traveling.

Poison Ivy/Oak

This very irritating skin rash, which appears two to three days after contact, can be completely relieved with homeopathic treatment. I have had very good results with **Sulphur 30c** for the very hot, itchy, oozy rash that is worsened by warm bathing and scratching, even though scratching feels good at the time. Sulphur has not been previously mentioned and it is easily obtained anywhere homeopathic remedies are sold. Consult the Directory on page 78 for a listing. Consider **Rhus toxicodendron 30c** if the Sulphur does not relieve the burning itch. Keep the patient cool. Keep her out of the sun, and give her a cool bath. Pat her body dry with a towel instead of rubbing the skin, which will irritate the rash and possibly spread it. Make a strong tea with dried or fresh **Calendula flowers** by adding one cup of flowers to a quart of hot water. Steep for five minutes, strain off the flowers and pour the remaining tea into the bath. **Baking soda** added to the bath water will also cool down the burning sensation of the itch. **Oatmeal baths** are a very effective, well-known old-time remedy for treating this ailment. *The Art of Health,* listed in the Directory, has an oatmeal bath bag specifically for treating the burning itch associated with poison oak and ivy. This can be a very annoying, uncomfortable condition. Do all that you can to make your child more comfortable. Dehydration will make the condition worse. Give your child plenty of cool drinks and don't forget to give lots of water. Keep her room cool, avoid tight clothing, and put cotton sheets on the bed to make her more comfortable.

Rashes

If it seems like your baby is red and blotchy most of the time, that's probably because he is. Babies have extremely sensitive skin, and something as simple as contact with bed linens can bring out tiny bumps. Drooling, especially connected with teething, can produce facial rashes on your baby's cheeks and chin. These eruptions are not serious. Apply a little **Calendula salve** to soothe and protect the area from moisture and chaffing. **Calendula cream** is also great for those rashes of undetermined origin that older children get. It's very soothing and many times will completely clear up the rash.

Your baby might experience prickly heat (small red spots on a flushed area of the skin, usually the groin) in hot, humid weather. Keep him cool when it's hot outside. Sponge him with cool water, dusting him off with a **cornstarch-based powder**, and dress him in cotton. A **baking soda bath** is cooling and brings comfort. Depending on the size of the bathtub, mix two tablespoons to one cup baking soda in the bath water, and let him soak for at least eight minutes.

Intertrigo is a skin rash that occurs where two areas of the skin rub together, notably in the neck crease, between the buttocks, in the armpits, and in the leg and arm creases. You can treat intertrigo the same way that you treat prickly heat.

Some babies will have allergic skin reactions, most commonly to cow's milk, wheat, citrus fruits, and chocolate. An allergic skin rash can show up in nursing babies when the mother is ingesting the troublesome foods. If you suspect food allergy as the cause of your child's rash, consult your naturopathic physician and request allergy testing to determine the cause of irritation.

Sinus Congestion

My children had chronic sinus congestion, which they gradually outgrew, but not until they were in their teens.

Frequently, stuffed-up and runny noses can be the result of intolerances or allergies to foods or other substances. The most common allergens, apart from foods, are pollen, dust, mold, cats, and dogs. The most common food intolerances are dairy, wheat, and, believe it or not, many kinds of fruit. If sinus congestion seems to be a persistent problem for your child, and is not due to a cold, consult your family physician and have your child tested for allergies. There are many ways of testing, using hair, blood, or urine. There are also many ways to treat allergies. Of course, the most natural way is to avoid or eliminate the substance causing the problem, but this isn't always the easiest way. There are many options nowadays, and it really isn't necessary for your child to suffer. Check with your naturopathic physician and come up with a plan that works for you and your child.

If your kids suffer from colds that produce sinus congestion as part of their symptoms, there are several treatments available for acute relief. Steam inhalation gives temporary relief. Place a vaporizer in the child's bedroom near her bed. Add some **vapor balm** to break up sinus congestion. There are homeopathics indicated for sinus congestion as well. For a cold that comes on after exposure to cold, damp air, with frequent sneezing and heavy, watery, irritating nasal discharge, use **Allium cepa 30c**. In the case where nasal secretions are watery and produce cold sores accompanied by sharp burning sensations of the mucus membranes of the nose, where the nose is blocked and sneezing does not bring relief, use **Arsenicum 30c**.

For sinus congestion, prepare the remedy by placing about 10 pellets in a glass of water, and give a spoonful of the solution every hour until symptoms are relieved.

There are several natural over-the-counter combination remedies for colds and sinus congestion available in the

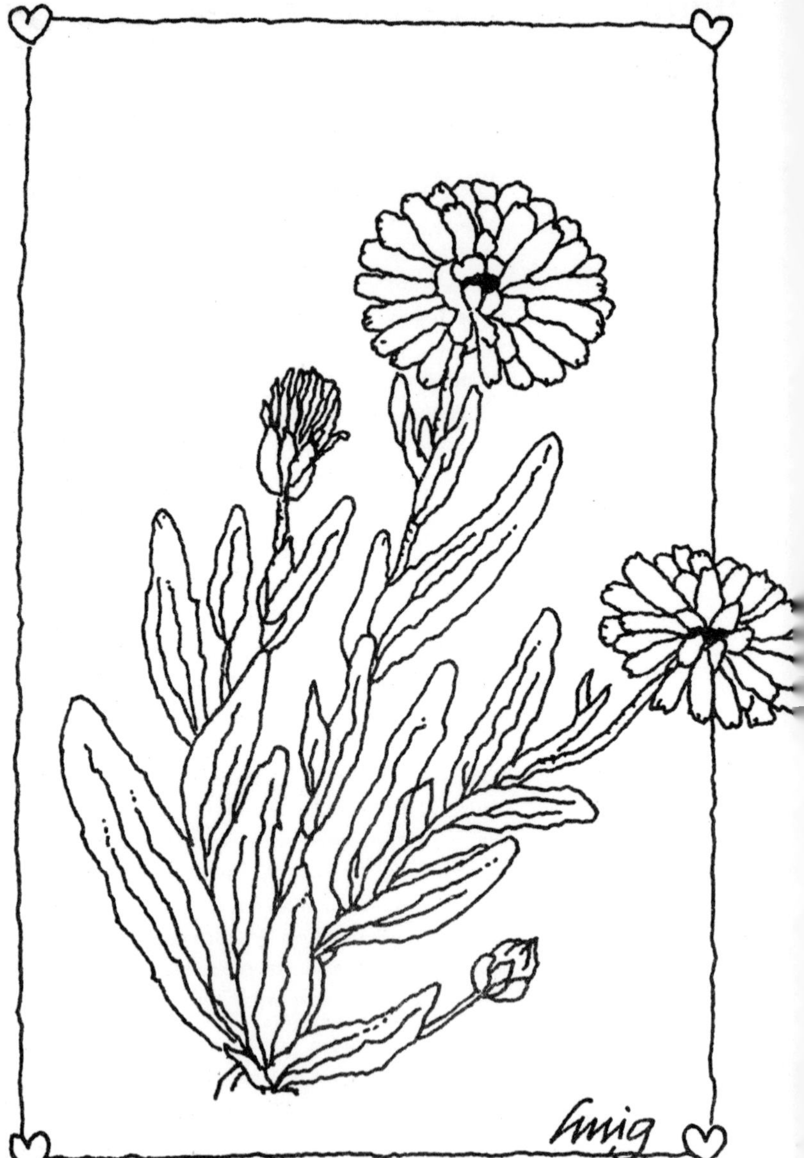

CALENDULA

Sinus congestion, continued

pill or liquid form. Look in the natural pharmaceutical section of your favorite healthfood store for these non-prescription remedies, or consult with your naturopathic physician, or call one of the companies listed in the Directory. Get these items ahead of time, so that when your child shows the first sign of feeling under the weather, you can treat her the before she gets really sick. Early treatment is the key to success in most cases.

Sleeplessness

A most unpleasant situation for all is a tired youngster who can't get to sleep. A massage accompanied by a lullaby calms both the mother and the child. Babies love back, tummy, and foot massage. It's a good idea to pick up a book on infant massage if this is an area you are unfamiliar or uncomfortable with. Usually a little back or foot massage will relax even the fussiest child. My oldest boy had an irritable disposition and was often difficult at bedtime. A back rub or foot massage always calmed him down. Turn off or dim the lights when massaging the young patient, or light a candle in a fire-safe container. Create an atmosphere of relaxation. If your little one isn't quite asleep after the massage, blow out the candle and tell a story in the dark. Most children love stories you make up, especially when told in the dark. This is a good way to get children to enjoy darkness rather than fear it.

If you feel it's necessary, there are a few homeopathic remedies to try. Use **Chamomilla 30c** for the fussy child who is impossible to please and complains too much. Then there is **Coffea 30c** for the agitated, wound-up kid who's spinning his wheels and is wide awake. **Arsenicum 30c** is for the very high-strung, restless, nervous child who is prone to fright. This child wants to keep getting out of bed after you have already said goodnight. He worries about things and is anxious.

Sleeplessness, continued

A warm washcloth placed on the back of his neck just before retiring is also helpful. If you want to give tea, **chamomile** is the best tea to help bring on sleep. A combination tea that contains chamomile and mint tastes a little better than just plain chamomile. If you're up to the task, a warm **chamomile, valerian, and lavender bath**, or just a foot bath with these herbs will soothe, calm, and relax your child.

Slivers and Stickers

Whenever your child gets a little something stuck under his skin or fingernail, think of **Silica 30c.** This is a great remedy whose nature it is to push things out of the body. One dose is usually enough. If you cannot pull the sticker out easily, first soak the area in a cup of **comfrey tea** or a bowl of hot water mixed with a few tablespoons of **Epsom salts.** This should make the skin soft enough to penetrate with a sterilized needle and cause little pain. If there is pus in the area, the comfrey tea will draw it out quickly.

Sore Throat

Keep your child warm, and well rested if she has a sore throat. Eliminate dairy and sugar from the diet. Usually the tonsils swell up and sometimes a fever and phlegm are present. This is clearly a case of inflammation. As described in the section entitled Inflammation, give the recommended herbs in pill or liquid form. Build up the immune system with **garlic**, **goldenseal,** and **Echinacea.** Add **vitamins A and C** to the regimen. Older children can gargle with **warm salt water;** use one teaspoon of salt to one cup of very warm water. There are some great homeopathic combination remedies specifically for sore throats that have worked very well for my family. The NF brand, formula **Pharyngin**, or the cell salt combination

Sore Throat, continued

simply titled *Sore Throat,* available in healthfood stores, always brought quick relief to my children. These remedies are available from any naturopathic physician and at many stores that carry natural remedies. Always keep some on hand, so that you can treat your little one at the onset of symptoms. They come in little pills that melt quickly when placed under the tongue, and are tasteless and non-irritating to the tender palate. I have never had to treat my children's sore throats with anything stronger than these remedies.

Combination tinctures for sore throats are also easy to use. Put about half a dropperfull in one of the following sore throat teas: **marshmallow, plantain,** or **catnip.** These all taste good and will not interfere with homeopathics. If you'd like to use straight non-combination remedies, the following are the most commonly used. **Aconite 30c** is given when symptoms come on suddenly after exposure to cold air, and the throat is red, dry, and swollen. **Belladonna 30c** is for the hot, very red sore throat that causes burning pain on swallowing, where the desire to swallow is frequent, and the child has a red, hot face with fever. Give a dose every half hour. If some relief doesn't come with two or three doses, stop or change the remedy. This is the general rule when treating acute conditions. If relief comes, stop giving the remedy and only repeat if the symptoms recur. **Zinc** or **slippery elm lozenges** are very helpful in soothing sore throats.

Sprains

Sprains can occur in many areas including arms, ankles, wrists, fingers and toes. You want to be sure nothing is broken. If you have any uncertainty, get an x-ray. A sprain is an injury to ligaments around a joint, causing pain, swelling, and skin discoloration. With a sprain there is usually no loss of mobility, as seen with a break, although it is frequently as painful, or more so. My favorite little skate boarder is an expert at treating his own sprained

Sprains, continued

ankles. The first step is to give **Arnica 30c** and repeat the remedy three to four times a day for the first two or three days. Then give **Hypericum 30c** if nerve damage is suspected. If there is bruising give **Ledum 30c.** Use either or both of these remedies three times a day, for about a week. After giving Arnica, ice and elevate the affected joint, then soak it in a warm **Epsom salts** bath at bedtime. If you have some **comfrey** leaves on hand, you can make a comfrey bath instead of using Epsom salts.

Topically apply **arnica** ointment if the skin is not broken. If the skin is broken, use **comfrey ointment**. A **comfrey compress** applied to the sprain overnight can speed recovery. Wrap ankles and wrists with an ace bandage during the day for support, and splint fingers. A very good supplement for healing ligaments is *Ligaplex* available from any naturopathic physician.

Sunburn

Sunburn is a growing concern for parents now that the ozone layer is thinning. Always protect young children from the sun. Sunscreen is definitely recommended but not enough. Always put a hat on young children who have little or no hair on their head. Put t-shirts on kids when they are swimming on hot sunny days. Keep babies in the shade and remember to give kids lots of water, so they won't get dehydrated from the sun. If your child does get a sunburn, give him a tepid bath with a cup of **baking soda** mixed into the water. This will cool the skin down and prevent peeling. Gently rub **Hypericum oil** on the skin and give homeopathic **Urtica Urens 30c** internally to relieve the pain of sunburn. **Aloe vera gel** will relieve the burning pain and heal the skin rapidly. If you have an Aloe plant, cut off a leaf, peel back the outer skin and generously swab the sunburned areas. The ready-to-use gel from a bottle is just as effective. Repeat this treatment twice a day until the pain has been relieved.

Teething

Most babies and toddlers have some irritation associated with teething. Common symptoms include irritability, sore gums, nasal discharge, drooling, diarrhea, and insomnia. **Chamomile tea** is very comforting and helps baby to fall asleep. Make a cup of tea by pouring boiling water on to one teaspoon of the dried herb in a mug. When the tea has cooled, put a clean baby washcloth in a bowl and pour the strained tea over it. Set the bowl in the refrigerator and when it's cold, squeeze out the washcloth a little and give it to baby to suck. Give older children a cup of the tea every few hours. Homeopathic **Chamomilla 3x or 6x** potency can be used freely during teething bouts. (*Note: this is a lower potency than we have been using previously for other conditions.)* In many areas this remedy is found under the name 'teething tablets'. This remedy worked very well for my children when they were babies, as well as when they getting twelve year molars and wisdom teeth.

Babies enjoy chewing on almost everything while teething. The pressure feels good and actually relieves the pain. Find a brightly colored, big-beaded, non-toxic, plastic or wooden necklace to wear around your neck. Your baby will be attracted to the colors and eager to chew on it while you are holding her.

Plastic teething rings are sold at any baby store as well as grocery stores. Store the teething ring in the refrigerator and when she gets fussy give it to her to chew on.

Warts

Warts are fun and easy to treat. As my oldest boy sat down to dinner one night, he began to antagonize his little brother with something scary on his hand, which turned out to be several warts growing on his fingers. Immediately after dinner we went for a walk to see if we could find some **dandelions**. The white sap from the stem and root are used as a topical remedy for warts. Pick some

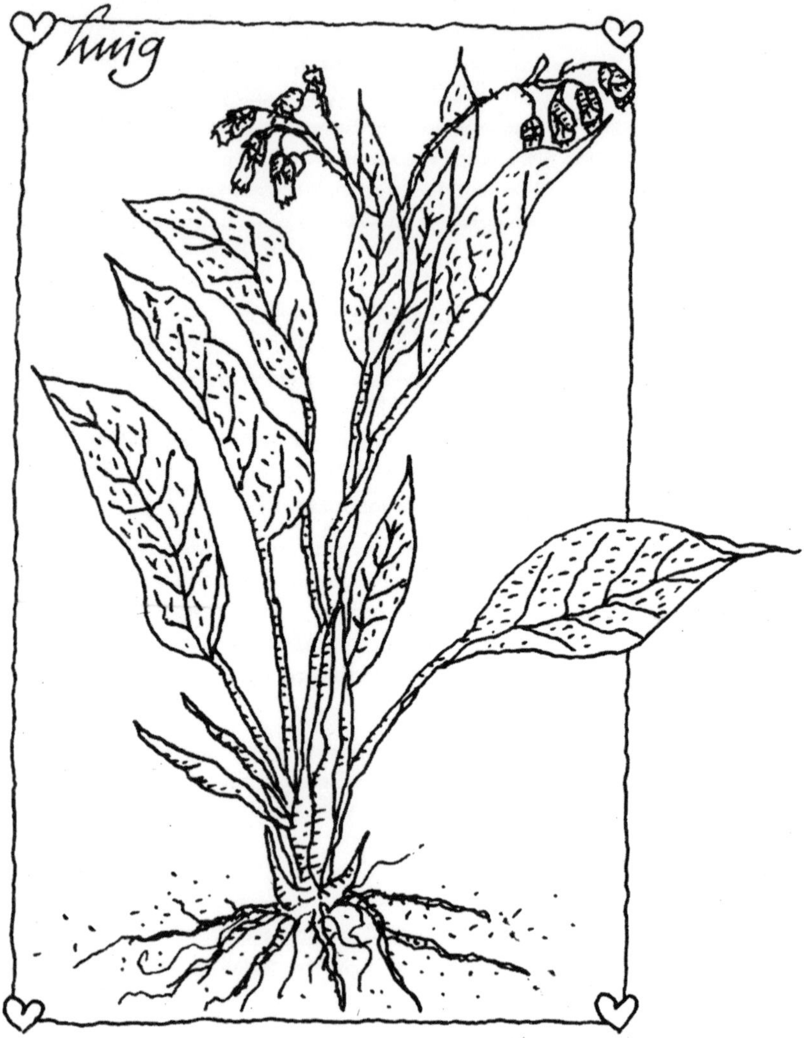

COMFREY

Warts, continued

leaves, or break off the root to expose the sap, and apply to the warts. Use this application daily. It may take a week or two for the warts to disappear. Your child will enjoy playing doctor in this way and can enjoy the success of healing himself.

Healing Words

There is nothing more powerful, soothing, and healing than the sound of the voice of someone you love. Use your voice to heal your children by verbally creating healing imagery through storytelling. All children love to hear stories you make up. When your child gets sick or injured, you can accelerate the healing process simply by telling her a story about a little child just like her, who has experienced a similar unfortunate situation.

Keep the story simple but the visual grand. Tell the story again and again. Unlike adults, children love to hear the same story over and over again. Repetition will ingrain healing energy into the body and mind of your precious little one.

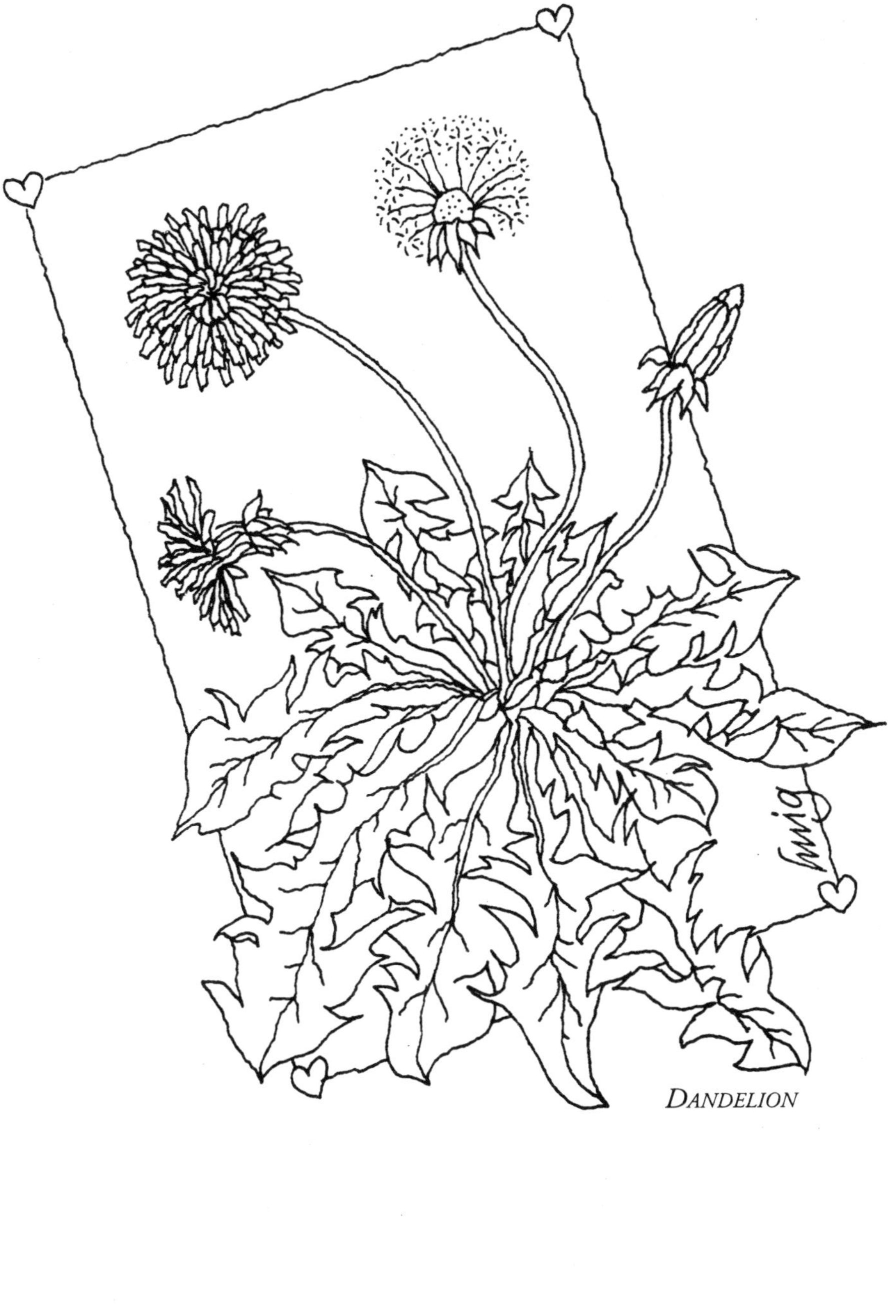

DANDELION

Glossary

ANTIBODIES: any of numerous protein molecules produced by B cells that play a primary immune system function.

BILIOUS: suffering caused by trouble with the bile or liver, producing peevish, irritable, or cranky behavior.

BIO-DYNAMIC: a method of gardening based on the study of mutual influences on living organisms. Emphasis is placed on observing the effects exerted on plants by their earthly and cosmic environment.

BOTANICAL: a medicine or drug made from the leaves, roots, bark, seeds, or flowers of plants.

CELL SALTS: twelve biochemical salts, tissue remedies, celloids, and cell salts that Schuessler, a German homeopathic physician, determined to be essential to the healthy functioning of the body.

COMPRESS: a cloth pad soaked in a hot herbal extract and applied to the painful area.

DECOCTION: tea made by boiling the botanical for a specified period of time, followed by straining or filtering.

DETOXIFICATION: the metabolic process by which toxins are changed into less toxic or more readily excretable substances.

HOMEOPATHY: a therapeutic medical science that holistically treats illness. The primary concept is to treat illness using minute doses of potentized substances.

HYDROTHERAPY: the use of water as a form of therapy to cure illness. It is a very powerful therapy and is of some use in virtually all diseases. Compresses, water packs, jet baths, steam treatments, and fomentations are just a few of the many water therapy techniques. This subject is too vast to cover, so you may wish to consult Drs. Boyle and Saine's excellent book, *Naturopathic Hydrotherapy* (Eclectic Medical Publishing, 14385 Southeast Lusted Road, Sandy, OR 97005)

MEDICINARY: pharmacy or medicine cabinet.

NATUROPATHIC MEDICINE: a drugless system of therapeutic medical science that comprises many natural healing techniques, including herbology, spinal and soft tissue adjustments, homeopathy, botanical medicines, hydrotherapy, acupuncture, nutritional guidance, and supplements (vitamins, glandular extracts, enzymes), and so on. Naturopathic physicians (indicated by N.D. after the name) are licensed to practice medicine in twelve states.

For more information, or to locate a Naturopath near you, contact the American Association of Naturopathic Physicians, 601 Valley Street., Ste #105, Seattle, WA 98102. (206) 298-0125.

In Britain, contact the General Council and Register of Naturopaths, Goswell House, 2 Goswell Road, Street, Somerset BA15 OJG. 01458-840 012.

POTENCY: the power, vitality, strength, or dynamis, which a homeopathic remedy possesses, often represented as a number attached to the remedy name either immediately before or after. The potency of a remedy comes as a result of the succussion step in the remedy preparation process. See also *potentize.*

POTENTIZE: the process of preparing a homeopathic remedy by repeated dilution with succussion (shaking). It may be said that potentization involves the transfer of information from a substance to the water in which it is dissolved.

POULTICE: a moist, warm, pasty mass folded inside a thin cloth and laid on inflamed skin to reduce inflammation, draw out infection, or act as a counterirritant. It promotes local circulation, causing collected pus and serum to either be absorbed into the system or brought to a head to discharge outwardly, thus giving relief.

PROPHYLAXIS: homeopathic remedy made from a disease.

TEPID: moderately warm, lukewarm.

TINCTURE: alcoholic or hydro-alcoholic solutions usually containing the active principles of botanicals in low concentrations.

'Children's minor illnesses and injuries can leave parents feeling helpless and worried. This little book shows the healing power of simple herbs, homeopathic medicines, foot baths, kind words, and rocking chairs. The remedies are as old as the hills, but Doctor Mom is a reliable health advisor for modern families.'

John Collins, N.D., Director of the Homeopathy Department at the National College of Naturopathic Medicine, Portland, OR.

'This is an excellent book of natural remedies for both kids and adults. I'm very excited to give this book to my patients. I've known Kathy for many years and have seen her raise all three of her kids with naturopathic medicine: Nature Heals.'

K.E. Edmisten, N.D. L.A.c.

'I met Kathy when I was a student in the National College of Naturopathic Medicine. At that time she was raising three small children as a single mother. Watching her children respond to these treatments and seeing the confidence she had about them was a tremendous experience for me. Kathy has described real life experience with natural treatments that work.'

David Greenspan, N.D.

'Kathy has always had a strong interest in natural healing and associated remedies. As one of her past naturopathic family physicians I saw her develop expertise in the use of a wide variety of natural medications. This book will serve as an excellent addition to the family home health library.'

Bruce Canvasser, N.D., President, N F Formulas, Wilsonville, OR.

‘As a midwife and naturopathic physician, I found Kathy’s book to be well researched, informative, and practical. As a mother of two, I think this book is perfect, with precise and easy to understand instructions. I have yet to come across another book like it.’

Katherine Zieman, N.D.,Licensed Midwife.

‘At home on the weekend, on your family vacation, or after 5:00 p.m. and there’s no doctor around? Well, now you can call on Doctor Mom’s Reference Guide to offer some help. If you have kids and want to use simple, safe, and effective natural remedies, buy this book. It’s the house call you’ve been wishing for.’

Tori Hudson, N.D., Professor of Gynecology, the National College of Naturopathic Medicine and Director of A Woman’s Time.

‘Dr. Mom’s is not only a joy to read, it is also a scientifically sound treasure chest of clinical pearls. Its readily accessible information is an invaluable resource for all mothers who wish to participate in their child’s healthcare.’

Laurie Regan, Ph.D, N.D.

NEW AGE BOOKS

THE ART AND SCIENCE OF PSYCHIC HEALING
—*Larry M. McDaniel* and *Phyllis G. McDaniel*

It is a book meant for anyone who is seeking personal development or improvement through psychic interpretations and divinations.

CHAKRA ENERGY MASSAGE—*Marianne Uhl*

This book guides you into the fascinating world of the energy body. Drawing on the knowledge gained by Foot Reflexology Massage, it introduces you to the Chakra Energy Massage. It provides detailed information on the healing effects of gemstones and the powers of fragrant essences, as well as the vibrations of primal tones and various colours, all of which can be employed to effectively enhance your work with the Chakras.
ISBN: 81-7822-004-0

THE INTUITIVE WAY—*Penney Peirce*

There's never been a book like The Intuitive Way! Comprehensive, easy, and entertaining to read, the author's no-nonsense approach inspires and instructs as no previous book on intuitive development has ever done.
ISBN: 81-7822-008-3

QUANTUM-TOUCH: THE POWER TO HEAL—*Richard Gordon*

Quantum-Touch represents a major breakthrough in the art of hands-on healing. Whether you are a complete novice, a professional chiropractor, physical therapist, body worker, healer, or other health professional, Quantum-Touch allows you a dimension of power in your work that heretofore has not seemed possible. Since the body already knows how to heal itself, the practitioner need only apply the energy to affected areas.
ISBN: 81-7822-009-1

UNCONDITIONAL BLISS (-Finding Happiness in the Face of Hardship)—*Howard Raphael Cushnir*

No matter how difficult life may be, you can still live in a state of radiant bliss—even if you're alone, sick, failed, and broke. This down-to-earth book shows us how. Based on universal spiritual principles, the message is profound and the method practical.
ISBN: 81-7822-013-x